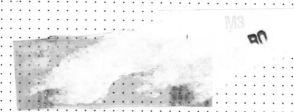

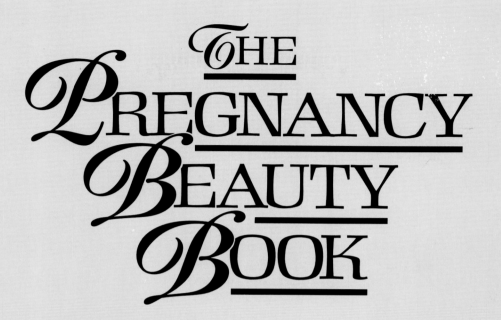

THE PREGNANCY BEAUTY BOOK

Heather Bampfylde

Foreword by
GAYLE HUNNICUTT

TIGER BOOKS INTERNATIONAL
LONDON

Design
Sally Strugnell

Editorial
Nicola Dent

Illustrations
Lawrie Taylor, Bernard Thornton Artists

Picture Research
Miriam Sharland

Picture Sources
Tony Stone Photolibrary - London
The Boots Company PLC
Mothercare
Lupe Cunha
The Hutchison Library
Pictor International
The Telegraph Colour Library
Colour Library Books Ltd
The Image Bank
St Mary's Hospital - London

No 3054
© 1992 Coombe Books
This 1992 edition published by
Tiger Books International PLC, London
All rights reserved
Printed in Singapore
ISBN: 1 85501 208 1

Contents

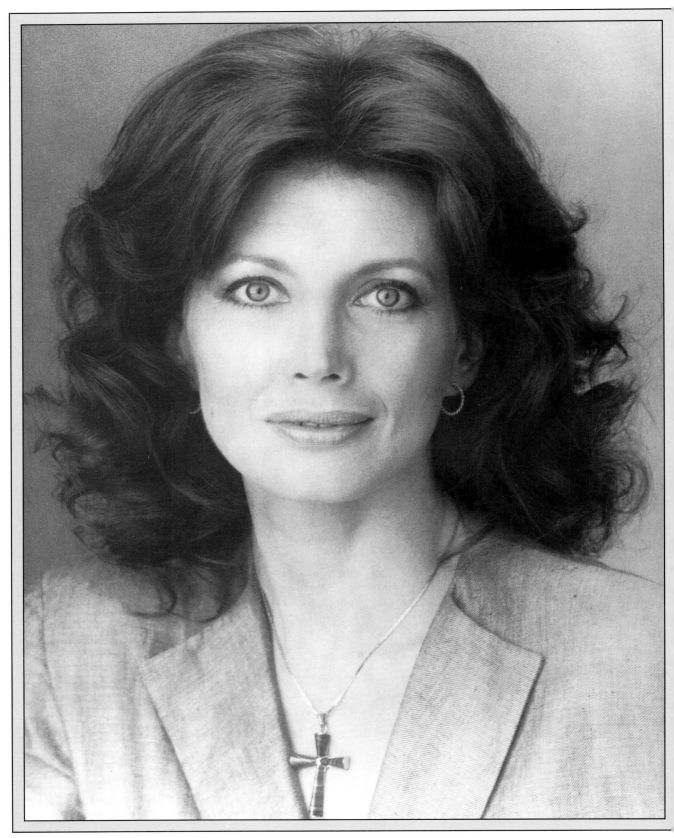

Foreword by Gayle Hunnicutt

This book is long overdue for the many women who did not receive beauty advice in their previous pregnancies and for those women who are embarking on the adventure of motherhood for the first time. Here is a book that advises not only on health matters but also on skincare, haircare, diet, exercise, relaxation and fashion.

Most books available tend to be medically orientated and ignore or only touch upon these important and morale-boosting aspects of personal care. During my last pregnancy I became so frustrated by this that I decided to write my own book, entitled Health and Beauty in Motherhood, in which I shared with my readers the invaluable information I have gained throughout the years from beauty and health care experts. I am delighted to see that there is now a new book on this subject which contains a wealth of practical and sympathetic advice for the expectant mother who wants to be physically and psychologically prepared for childbirth and motherhood.

Looking good at this important time in your life can help you to enjoy your pregnancy, increase your self-confidence and gain an improved body-image. Remember, you do not have to look frumpy, overweight or unattractive just because you are pregnant.

Women who work will find the book especially useful as there is advice on nutritious snacks which can be taken into the office with them, and also advice on how to cook easy, healthy meals at home. Beating morning sickness, backache and other pregnancy-related problems is important to working women who cannot afford to take too much time off work and who need to feel their best,

both mentally and physically, to meet the challenges of the job.

How to stay beautiful and avoid stretch marks, varicose veins and excessive weight gain are also featured. All these conditions are preventable. If allowed to happen, they may stay with you for the rest of your life, so it is best to take positive action to avoid them.

By following the guidelines for a healthy diet laid down in the book, you can feel better throughout your pregnancy and help to ensure that you have a healthy baby. Nothing is more important at this stage of your life than understanding and following the rules of good nutrition.

By exercising sensibly and regularly, you will be stronger and better able to cope with labour. You will also reduce the possibility of a Caesarean section, a prolonged delivery and tearing. Your body will regain its pre-pregnancy shape quicker and more easily, and you may actually find that your figure is better than ever, thanks to the good habits you have adopted in pregnancy.

The book has an easy-to-follow month-by-month guide to exercise, diet and beauty, which means that you can readily find the information you require at any stage in your pregnancy. The final sections on coming home with your new baby and getting your figure back to normal will help you adjust to the new demands and joys of motherhood.

I look back on my own two pregnancies with tremendous affection. I looked better and felt greater contentment than at any other time in my life. I feel sure that with the help of The Pregnancy Beauty Book, you will do the same.

Gayle Hunnicutt

Get fit and healthy for pregnancy

Get fit for pregnancy

Even before you discover that you are pregnant you can do a lot to ensure that you have a healthy baby and a happy, easy pregnancy. If you want to *look* good and *feel* good, it is worth getting fit for pregnancy and practising some preconceptual care. This means actively preparing yourself for pregnancy even before conception. It might entail a few changes in your lifestyle – like eating a more healthy, wholefoods diet, giving up smoking and alcohol, or embarking on a gentle exercise programme. It is mostly a matter of common sense.

If you are already pregnant, don't worry – it is better to start now than not at all. But it does make good sense to start living a healthier life three to six months before conception takes place. The fetus is at its most vulnerable during the early weeks of pregnancy when its vital organs are developing – usually before your pregnancy is even confirmed. This healthier way of living applies to your partner, too. You want his sperm to be as healthy as your egg. It may be affected by poor diet, pollution, drugs, smoking, alcohol or toxic metals such as lead. The fitter and stronger you both are, the better your chances of having an enjoyable pregnancy, a trouble-free delivery and a healthy bouncing baby at the end of it all.

Your environment

This may affect your health and that of your baby, too, so take a few simple precautions both before and during pregnancy to help protect you both from any ill effects and environmental hazards.

Your workplace may be potentially hazardous, especially if you are working with chemicals or machines that emit low levels of radiation. A report by the UK Chemical Industries Association in 1984 recognized the link between certain chemicals and birth defects in the babies of mothers who worked with them. As the risk is greatest even before you know you are pregnant, you should either change your job or transfer to another department if you are worried. The same applies to your husband as his sperm may be damaged, too, by exposure to dangerous chemicals.

New research in Canada and Holland may have discovered a link between birth defects, stillbirths and miscarriages and women who work with VDUs (visual display units) and data processing machines. However, more research is required before any definite conclusions can be drawn.

Lead is another environmental hazard and difficult to avoid in some cases. It has been linked with birth defects and a high incidence of stillbirths. Unfortunately, it is present in tap water, car exhaust fumes, cigarette smoke, newsprint and some paints. So avoid dense traffic, use lead-free paints when decorating and try to drink bottled mineral water if your house has lead pipes. At least, draw off a couple of gallons of water before drinking or boiling it. Eating more calcium-rich foods such as milk, cheese and green vegetables, and zinc in the form of meat and seafood may help absorb lead and reduce this toxic metal to more acceptable levels in your body.

Alcohol is another potential hazard to your unborn baby, and may cause birth handicaps known collectively as Fetal Alcohol Syndrome. Doctors still don't know what constitutes a safe, acceptable level of drinking but it seems that even a moderate amount of alcohol taken in the earliest weeks of the baby's development could produce low birth weight, a slow rate of development and limb, facial and joint deformities. If you choose to drink, keep it to a minimum – perhaps for special occasions only and always with a meal so that the alcohol will be absorbed more slowly into your bloodstream. Better still, give up drinking altogether at least for the duration of your pregnancy.

Smoking and its dangers are well-known and it is preferable that you give up smoking before you conceive rather than waiting for your pregnancy to be confirmed. When you smoke, the toxic chemicals

If you take steps to improve your lifestyle now before you conceive, you can look forward with confidence to your pregnancy. You will help eliminate any pregnancy-related health problems and maximize your chances of an easier delivery and giving birth to a healthy baby.

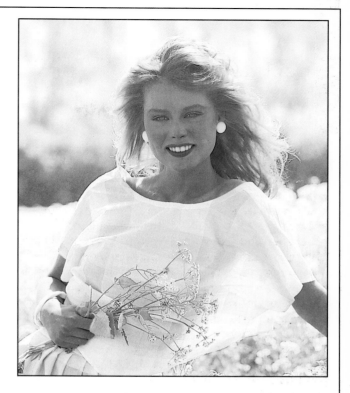

enter your bloodstream and are passed via the placenta to your baby. They can damage the placenta itself and interfere with the flow of nutrients and oxygen to the baby. Smoking can also predispose you to a higher risk of miscarrying. Ask yourself whether it is worth the risk, and whether your baby should have the right to a healthy environment inside you – you can choose, she can't.

Relax

Reducing any stress in your life and making time to relax are very important if you are hoping to conceive and wish to achieve a full-term pregnancy. Make time each day for some conscious relaxation – meditation and yoga are especially beneficial. Flaking out in front of the TV after a hard day's work is not necessarily relaxing if your mind is still whirling with the day's events and crises. Relaxation exercises and deep breathing for just 10 minutes a day will help you find inner tranquility and leave you feeling refreshed and revitalized.

Exercising your choices

The fitter and stronger your body, the more likely you are to sail through pregnancy, have a quicker delivery and a healthy baby. Regular exercise will help your body prepare itself for the stresses of pregnancy and if you are reasonably fit and slim before you conceive you have a better chance of staying that way throughout your pregnancy and regaining your figure quickly after the birth. You need to develop muscle control and endurance for the ordeal of labour; strong back and abdominal muscles for bearing the growing weight of the baby in the last months; and strong pelvic floor muscles for an easier birth and a diminished risk of tearing.

Don't embark on a really tough exercise programme if you are unused to strenuous physical activity. Take it gently and don't strain or push yourself too far, too fast. Choose a form of exercise

that you enjoy – it may be jogging, cycling, swimming, aerobics or weight-training. Exercise at least four times a week for 30 minutes each session. You will be able to continue with your exercise programme well into your pregnancy although you may have to make a few changes as the baby gets bigger and heavier. During the later months it is best to follow a special pregnancy programme of antenatal exercises (see page 56). To be on the safe side, check with your doctor that your usual routine is quite safe.

Your health

If you want a baby you should try to be as healthy as possible. If you are at all worried about your own health or that of your husband, you could have a complete medical check-up. Most important of all, you should ascertain whether you have ever had German measles and built up a rubella immunity. A simple blood test will tell you if you are not sure. Contracting rubella in the early months of pregnancy may result in your baby being born deaf, blind or with a damaged heart. Don't take the risk. Find out and be immunized immediately if you have no immunity. Then wait three months before trying to conceive – use contraception during this time.

Get fit and healthy for pregnancy

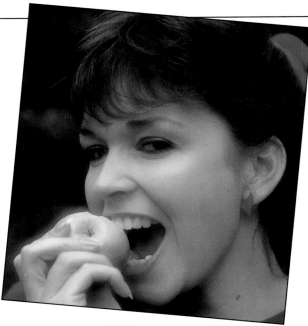

Include a variety of fresh fruit and vegetables in your diet; natural wholefoods are better than processed foods, which often contain additives.

Healthy diet

The food you eat in this preconceptual period will set the pattern for your pregnancy diet to some extent. It will establish new, healthier eating habits which will benefit you for life and which you can pass on to your child. Good-quality wholefoods with nothing added or taken away form the basis of good health and beauty. They can prevent many pregnancy-associated ailments such as morning sickness and varicose veins, and will make your skin glow, your hair look really glossy and give you energy, too. They also provide the essential nutrients that your baby will need for growth and development, and for protection against infection and pollution. It is important that nutrients are available from the exact moment of conception to enable the cells to carry out their specific functions and nourish the baby.

You will need some of the following fresh, unrefined foods. Try to vary them and make your diet as interesting and diverse as possible. Choose from fresh meat, poultry, offal, game, fish and shellfish, fruit, vegetables, beans and pulses, whole-grain cereals, eggs, low-fat cheese and yoghurt. Try to avoid processed convenience foods that are laced with chemical additives. You an check their content by reading the labels carefully before buying. Many additives are potentially harmful to the health of a tiny baby, especially a fetus. Some are now being linked with birth defects and are cited as contributory factors in causing hyperactivity in small children. Watch out especially for the following additives with the E-prefix: E123 (amaranth); E124 (tartrazine); E249 (potassium nitrite); E250 and E251 (sodium nitrite and nitrate); E320 (BHA) and E321 (BHT); and E621 (monosodium glutamate).

So what should you eat?

The daily nutrients you need for the maintenance of good health are:
Protein to build your baby's tiny body. So eat fish,

meat, poultry, cheese, eggs, milk, yoghurt, whole-grain cereals, wholemeal bread, beans and pulses (lentils, split peas) and nuts.

Carbohydrates to provide the energy to meet the needs of your growing baby. These include whole-grain cereals, wholemeal bread, brown rice, wholemeal pasta, muesli and starchy vegetables.

Vitamins for the healthy development of your baby. If you eat a varied healthy diet, it need not be necessary to take vitamin supplements, but a deficiency of any one vitamin can affect your baby's health so make sure that you are getting some of the following:

Vitamin A in fish liver oils, kidney, liver, eggs and dairy produce, dark green vegetables, yellow fruit and vegetables and dried apricots.

Vitamin B-complex, especially B6, B12 and folic acid. Eat whole-grain cereals and bread, liver, brewers yeast, dark green leafy vegetables, meat, fish, eggs, cheese, avocados and bananas.

Vitamin C to protect your baby against infection. Eat citrus fruits, peppers, tomatoes, strawberries, blackcurrants, baked potatoes and dark green leafy vegetables.

Vitamin D for your baby's bones. Eat oily fish, milk, cheese and eggs.

Vitamin E for healthy red blood cells. Eat whole-grain cereals, vegetable oils, avocados.

Minerals for your health and your baby's development. In particular, you need **calcium** from cheese, milk, and yoghurt for building bones and teeth; **zinc** from seafoods, meat, liver and eggs for healthy cell division and fertility; and **iron** from liver, eggs and dark green vegetables for healthy red blood cells. You also need fats (preferably in the form of vegetable oils and low-fat cheese and yoghurt) and dietary fibre, as will be discussed later.

Caffeine is a substance found in coffee, tea and Coca-Cola. Although there is no absolute proof that too much caffeine can harm your baby, some doctors suspect that this may be the case, so you should cut down on the cuppas you drink. Limit your tea and coffee consumption to, say, three cups per day and cut out Coke altogether which is loaded with sugar and has no place in a healthy diet. Drink decaffeinated coffee or, better still, increase the number of fresh juices you drink – they are a valuable source of vitamins and minerals.

The Pill can deplete your own supply of zinc and vitamin B6 – both valuable nutrients for a trouble-free pregnancy and healthy baby. Although you can take supplements to compensate for this or ensure that you receive the recommended amounts from your new varied diet, it is a good idea to stop taking the Pill at least three months before you plan to conceive. Use some other form of contraception while your body is readjusting to its normal menstrual cycle.

Drugs should never be taken unless prescribed by your doctor – even aspirin, cough mixture, pain relievers and antibiotics. However, these may be prescribed right at the beginning of your pregnancy before it is even confirmed. So if you are planning to have a baby and are no longer using contraception and are ill or have a medical condition that requires treatment with drugs, tell your doctor and ask which

ones are safe to use. Try to do without them for any minor ailments like colds, indigestion and headaches.

Are you fit for pregnancy?

If you actively practise all the measures outlined above you have the best possible chance of having a healthy child. But even if you are already pregnant and did not know about preconceptual care, as long as you eat a varied diet and give up drinking and smoking you have nothing to worry about. It's never too late to start leading a healthier life so change the habits of a lifetime *now*. You will be amazed at how much better you will feel and the beauty spin-offs, too, as you will see in the coming chapters.

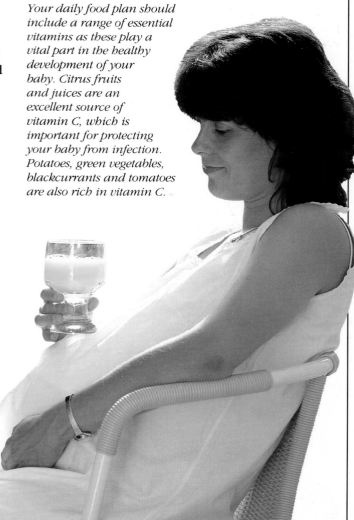

Your daily food plan should include a range of essential vitamins as these play a vital part in the healthy development of your baby. Citrus fruits and juices are an excellent source of vitamin C, which is important for protecting your baby from infection. Potatoes, green vegetables, blackcurrants and tomatoes are also rich in vitamin C.

Recognize the early symptoms

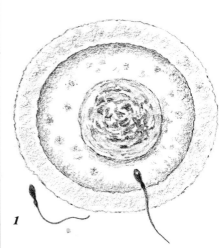

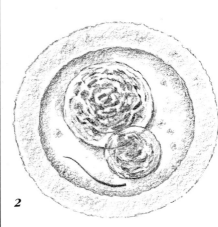

You

Your pregnancy is calculated from the first day of your last period even though conception usually takes place two weeks afterwards. During this first month you are probably unaware that you are pregnant although you may be hoping that this is the case. The first sign of pregnancy is a missed period and this will not be noticed until the fourth week. Even then you might just think that it is late and not realize that you are already pregnant.

However, by the fifth or sixth week some physical signs will be manifesting themselves:-

1 Your breasts may feel tender and fuller than usual due to hormonal changes deep within your body as it prepares for breastfeeding. By the sixth week – about 10 days after you miss your period – small nodules known as Montgomery's tubercules may appear on the dark areolae around your nipples. The network of blood vessels on your breasts may also be more noticeable than usual.

2 You may want to pass water more frequently than usual and even wake up in the night to do so.

3 You may feel more tired than you normally do as your body starts to adjust to pregnancy.

These are the classic early symptoms of pregnancy and the indicators of great changes that are going to take place inside your body in the coming months.

A simple pregnancy test will ascertain whether you are pregnant and may be carried out from the tenth day after conception onwards. This consists of a simple urine test. Your doctor or clinic will send off a urine sample for testing or you can buy a home-testing kit over the counter in a chemist or drugstore. Be sure to test the first-passed urine of the day before drinking anything in the morning. An early drink might dilute the pregnancy hormones. To test it yourself you must mix the amount of urine

1 *Having reached the fallopian tube, one of the sperm penetrates the ripened egg, which has been released by one of the ovaries.*

2 *The head of the sperm, the gene-carrying nucleus, separates from the tail and fuses with the egg's nucleus.*

3 *The egg divides into two cells as the chromosomes of the two nuclei pair off and development begins.*

4 *Cell division continues as the egg makes its journey along the fallopian tube towards the uterus.*

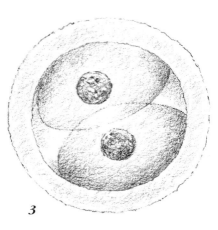

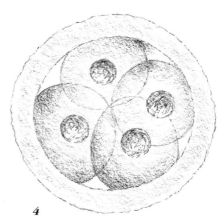

specified on the kit instructions with the chemicals provided. This is usually done in a test tube. It is shaken and then left for about two hours before checking for signs of pregnancy. A dark ring is a positive result and can be viewed in the mirror provided. If there is no HCG hormone in your urine to provide this result, then either you are *not* pregnant or you have carried out the test too early. If this happens, and the result is negative, don't be discouraged. If your period still does not arrive, test again and this time it may be positive. Congratulations!

Your baby

Your child's genetic make-up is decided at the moment of conception at or around the time of ovulation. The ripened egg is released from one of your ovaries and passes through a fallopian tube towards the uterus. Fertilization takes place when one of your partner's sperm fuses with the egg. As sperm can survive in your body for up to seven days, intercourse does not have to take place at the exact time of ovulation for fertilization to occur although it will obviously increase your chance of success.

Now the process of cell division begins and when the fertilized egg finally reaches the uterus it embeds itself in the wall and is nourished by a system of blood vessels in the uterus. Already, the placenta, its unique life-support system, is beginning to form in readiness to take over the job of supplying oxygen and nutrients to the growing baby.

But at the moment your baby is still a cluster of rapidly dividing cells with a cavity that will become the amniotic sac within which the baby will float and an inner cell mass which will become the fetus itself. By the fifth week since the date of your last period, an embryo is forming, with a spine and two lobes of a rudimentary brain. At this time it is about 2mm/one-tenth of an inch long. By the sixth week it has a head and trunk and even tiny limbs in the making.

These first few weeks are a critical time for the embryo as they are a period of rapid growth and development when its brain and limbs are forming. So it is very important that you eat a healthy diet supplying all the nutrients it needs for normal development. You can also provide a healthy environment within your body by not smoking or drinking alcohol and by endeavouring to stay away from toxic and harmful fumes and metals.

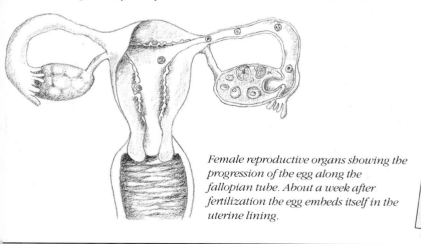

Female reproductive organs showing the progression of the egg along the fallopian tube. About a week after fertilization the egg embeds itself in the uterine lining.

Change your lifestyle now

If you have not been following the general principles of preconceptual care it is not too late to start now. Here's what you do:

1 Give up smoking.

2 Stop drinking alcohol.

3 Eat a healthy, varied diet of fresh ingredients and wholefoods.

4 Check that you are not taking any harmful drugs. Ask your doctor for advice.

5 Embark on a gentle exercise programme to get your muscles well-toned and your body into shape for what is to come.

6 Try to relieve any stressful areas in your life and learn to relax and unwind. Above all, don't worry about the pregnancy. It is a happy time when you can enjoy all the changes taking place within your body.

Establish the right pregnancy skincare routine

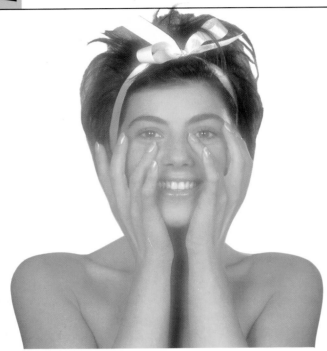

Pregnancy is the best beauty treatment your skin can have, or, at least, that's what most women find. You may notice a change in your skin as early as the first month as the pregnancy hormones get to work inside your body. If you are lucky you will look radiant with clear, glowing, healthy skin. Any blemishes or oily patches normally disappear and your skin may look better than it has ever done before. However, a minority of women do seem to experience skin problems – excessive oiliness or dryness depending on the stage of pregnancy they have reached.

Developing a good, effective skincare routine that suits your skin type is very important to keep skin smooth and moist. You can get into good habits now that will last a lifetime and will always stand you in good stead. Beautiful healthy skin is usually the result of meticulous, regular care rather than just good fortune. It's not hard work and need not take too long to achieve each day – just a few minutes when you get up in the morning and before you go to bed at night.

Basic rules for healthy skin

1   Never go to bed wearing make-up. It can clog and block the pores in your skin leading to spots.
2   Always cleanse thoroughly at night to remove all traces of stale make-up, grime, dirt and pollutants.
3   Cleanse in the morning before applying your make-up so that your skin is really fresh and clean and to get rid of any oiliness that may have accumulated during the night.
4   After cleansing always use a gentle toner or freshener to close the pores and remove all traces of cleanser. It will leave your skin feeling tingly, squeaky clean.
5   Always moisturize thoroughly to prevent dryness and keep skin moist and smooth – this will help stave off the ageing process and keep your skin looking youthful. Although you cannot add moisture to your skin, you can prevent it losing its natural moisture.
6   Use the right products for your skin type and change them if necessary to suit your skin during pregnancy.

The secret of your pregnancy skincare beauty routine is to adapt it to changing conditions as it is unlikely that your skin will stay the same throughout the whole nine months. Start off by analyzing your skin type.

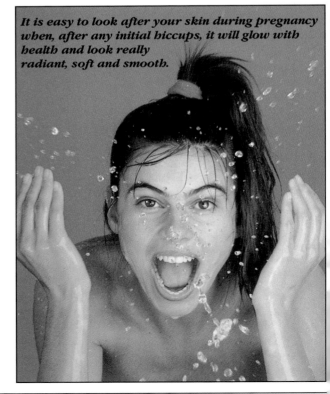

It is easy to look after your skin during pregnancy when, after any initial hiccups, it will glow with health and look really radiant, soft and smooth.

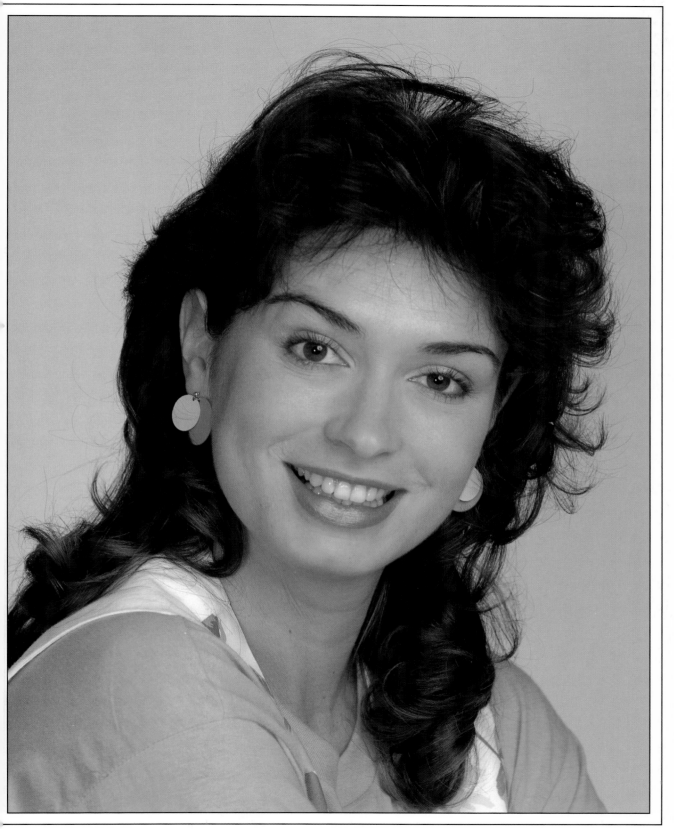

Establish the right pregnancy skincare routine

1 Dry skin

Most women find that their skin gets drier in the first trimester of pregnancy due to increased oestrogen in their bodies. It is easily recognizable as the skin feels taut, dry and flaky, especially after cleansing. Tiny lines round the eyes and mouth may appear and, also, your skin may be more sensitive than usual.

Skincare: cleanse gently with a mild cleanser – liquid or soap. Rinse off with warm water and pat dry. Some experts recommend applying a thin film of oil to the face before cleansing to help seal in the skin's natural moisture which harsh soaps can strip away. Use a mild, not an astringent, toner and afterwards moisturize deeply to nourish your skin and seal in any moisture that may escape into the air.

This is essential in cold weather or hot sunshine which are both very drying to the skin. Another way to help keep skin moist is to keep a humidifier in your bedroom or living room to add moisture to the air. Central heating and air conditioning are both natural enemies of good skin and can contribute to dryness through dehydrating the skin.

Use a light moisturizer in the morning under make-up and a rich moisturizer at night. A water-in-oil emulsion is best for dry skin as it forms a thin, protective layer of oil on the surface to prevent moisture evaporation. You can also treat yourself to a specially formulated dry skin face pack once a week. If your skin tends to be very sensitive, use hypo-allergenic products minus the fragrances which may irritate. Cleansing with a special super-fatted soap will also help add moisture.

2 Oily skin

Later on in your pregnancy you may get an oil problem when the progesterone levels in your body are higher than usual. After the birth, your skin will probably revert to normal but in the meantime you need to know how to look after it. It is unlikely that

Analyse your skin type
In order to treat your skin correctly you have to get to know it. Here is a basic guide to help you with identification. To examine your skin, cleanse thoroughly and study it closely in a magnifying or shaving mirror. Be positive and critical and do not gloss over any imperfections.

Type	Characteristics	Its nature	Location
Normal	Moist, smooth and free from blemishes and problems. No dry or excessively oily patches	Although called normal, it is rare, and usually the preserve of young women	All over face and neck
Oily	Skin looks shiny and feels greasy, is prone to spots, blackheads and blocked pores, even acne	Found in all ages, especially young. Sebaceous glands over produce sebum, especially during hormonal changes. Good for older women as cuts down risk of wrinkles	Centre panel of face – nose, forehead, chin, also back and chest
Dry	Dry, flaky and tight. Sensitive and prone to lines and broken veins. May look dull or crêpey	Skin does not produce enough oil and thus its moisture evaporates leaving it dry. Wind, sun, air conditioning, heating and harsh soaps worsen the condition	Cheeks, throat and around eyes
Sensitive	Easily irritated and prone to broken veins and redness. May have flaky patches and be allergic to certain substances	Skin may be dry or oily and reacts adversely to extremes of heat and cold, harsh soaps and detergents	All over face and neck or localised
Combination	Oily patches, especially in central panel, and dry patches, usually on cheeks	Most common skin type which necessitates two different types of skincare – creams for dry *and* oily skin	Cheeks, throat and sides of forehead are dry; nose, chin and middle of forehead are oily

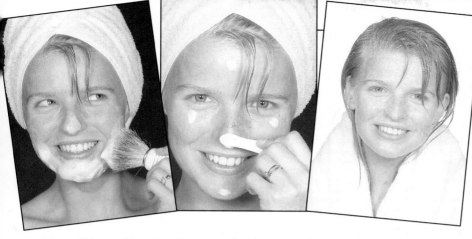

Cleansing, moisturizing and toning should become an essential part of your daily routine, when you get up and before going to bed. Choose the products that suit your skin type.

your skin will be uniformly oily – usually the central panel through your forehead, nose and chin is oily – while your cheeks may remain quite dry. To test for oiliness, blot your face with a tissue immediately after waking before cleansing. Any oily patches will show up as shiny areas on the tissue. Pores may look enlarged and get clogged, and there is often a tendency to spots, blackheads and blemishes – indeed, the overall effect is rather coarse. Of course, not all women get oily skin and the chances are that if you are naturally inclined to oiliness and blemishes, that pregnancy will clear it up and improve your skin tone and texture.

Skincare: cleanse at least twice a day, preferably with a soap or cleansing bar and water. This is very important to keep the skin clean and to ensure that pores do not get blocked. Use a freshener or toner afterwards, applied on cotton wool pads, to tighten the skin and close the pores. The new thinking is that you should not use too astringent and harsh a toner on oily skin. Although this is traditionally recommended, it may, in fact, exacerbate the problem. The more excess oil removed, the worse the condition may become. For drying the skin to remove oil can also have the opposite effect of stimulating the sebaceous glands to replace the lost oil.

Even though your skin is already oily, you must moisturize it with a very light moisturizer, the oil-in-water kind is best. Apply gently and evenly all over your face. To keep skin really healthy and get rid of any blackheads, you should exfoliate it twice a week. This helps remove the dead skin cells on the skin's surface, usually with a specially formulated abrasive product.

3 Normal skin

Although we all want this, not many of us get it – unblemished, smooth, moist skin with an even tone and colour and neither dry nor oily patches. You might be fortunate and find that pregnancy has this effect on your skin but you will still need to look after it to keep it that way.

Skincare: cleanse with a gentle cleanser, freshen and moisturize twice a day. You don't need a deep-action moisturizer – a light one will do.

Diet and your skin

The food you eat directly affects your skin. In fact, its appearance is a reflection of your inner state of health. During pregnancy you should be eating a varied highly nutritious diet which supplies all the nutrients you need for optimum health, and this is one of the reasons why many women's skins look so marvellous and radiant. Many skin problems stem from bad diet as well as inadequate skincare. The best food for your skin is fresh, unrefined and with nothing added nor taken away – fruit, vegetables, whole-grain cereals, vegetable oils, beans and pulses, eggs, yoghurt, milk, cheese, fish, shellfish, meat and poultry (unless you are vegetarian, of course). The foods that are enemies of good skin include cakes, crisps, biscuits, sweets, chocolate, sugar and other over-refined foods which add little in the way of nutrients and contribute to toxic wastes in the body.

A high-fibre diet not only helps prevent constipation, varicose veins and piles but it also benefits your skin by eliminating wastes and toxins from your body. Daily helpings of wholemeal bread, muesli with bran, fresh fruit and vegetables will all keep skin looking healthy. Drinking plenty of mineral water, say, five or six glasses a day, will also detoxify your skin, improve its circulation and help avoid cellulite (this is the build-up of fatty deadened tissue that often accumulates on hips, thighs and the upper arms in pregnancy).

Establish the right pregnancy skincare routine

Vitamins are vital: these organic substances are essential for your skin's health and beauty. You need:
1   **Vitamin A** to regulate the functioning of the skin's glands and control oiliness. Lack of it can cause dryness, scaliness and enlarged pores. Good sources are yellow fruits and vegetables, carrots, dark green leafy vegetables, fish oils, eggs and liver.
2   **Vitamin B-complex** aids skin circulation and controls excessive oiliness. It has been discovered that many skin problems may be linked with a deficiency of vitamin B in the diet. A daily 15ml/1 tablespoon of brewers yeast, or the equivalent amount of tablets if you dislike the flavour, will be beneficial. You should ensure that you get sufficient B-complex vitamins from eating whole-grain cereals, liver, leafy green vegetables, nuts, fish, poultry, eggs and legumes.
3   **Vitamin C** is essential for healthy skin collagen – the network of protein fibres that gives skin its resilience, firmness, youthfulness and elasticity. It protects these fibres and helps prevent broken veins by keeping the capillaries that supply nutrients to the cells strong and healthy. Citrus fruits, strawberries, peppers, dark green leafy vegetables, tomatoes and baked potatoes all provide vitamin C.
4   **Vitamin E** slows down your skin's natural ageing process as well as stimulating circulation. Because it is a natural antioxidant it helps prevent cell damage, form new cells and improve cell respiration. Deficiencies lead to premature wrinkling. Good sources are wheatgerm, green leafy vegetables, whole-grain cereals, avocados and vegetable oils.

Minerals are marvellous: some minerals contribute to your skin's natural beauty.
1   **Iodine** helps prevent your skin becoming coarse or wrinkled. Using iodized sea salt probably ensures the recommended daily dose, but it is also found in shellfish and fish, onions and legumes.
2   **Selenium** slows down the ageing process in your skin and helps keep the tissues elastic. Garlic, brewers yeast, liver, eggs, tomatoes and broccoli all contain this mineral.

3   **Sulphur** is vital for healthy skin and tissue respiration. Deficiencies can lead to scaliness. Eggs, green vegetables, fish and beans are good sources.
4   **Zinc** is probably the most important mineral of all for healthy skin. It is required for collagen synthesis and building cells. It is particularly useful in pregnancy for preventing stretch marks as we shall see. Women who have been on the Pill may suffer from zinc deficiency so it may be a good idea to take a supplement just to be on the safe side. However, a diet that includes seafood, meat, whole-grain cereals and legumes should provide adequate amounts.

Your skin and the sun

If you are pregnant during a long, hot summer you will have to take special care of your skin as the sun can not only burn you but it may also bring about changes in the skin's pigmentation and any damage may be intensified. The sun's ultra-violet rays are probably your skin's worst enemy and certainly the fastest, most efficient way to age it prematurely. Although they promote a healthy-looking golden tan, they do untold damage by breaking down the supportive collagen fibres and causing them to cross-link. This creates fine lines and wrinkles in time, especially around the eyes and mouth. Eventually the skin loses its firmness and elasticity and it literally ages. It also suffers from moisture loss and therefore it is essential to protect it at all times in the sun.

This does not mean to say that you should stay out of the sun altogether but you should take adequate precautions to minimize any sun-damage. In this way you can tan safely and painlessly. You may not go a deep leathery bronze but you will have a glamorous golden colour. If you are heavily pregnant you probably won't want to stay too long in the sun anyway as you may feel uncomfortable. Here are the golden rules to tanning safely:

1   Build up your tan gradually

Don't spend hours lying in the sun on the first hot summer's day. Take it easy and slowly, especially if you are on holiday in a sunspot. Build up from just 30 or 45 minutes' exposure on the first day to several hours at the end of the week, gradually lengthening the time outside. This is essential if you are naturally fair-skinned and inclined to burn easily.

2   Avoid the hottest time of the day

The hours between 11am and 3pm are the most

dangerous when the sun's rays are at their most powerful and intense, so stay out of the sun in the middle of the day and confine your sunbathing to early morning and late afternoon. Sit in the shade and sip a cooling, refreshing fruit juice instead. Remember that the nearer you are to the Equator the more damaging the sun will be.

3 Always wear a sunscreen

A good sunscreen will help filter out the harmful burning rays and promote a light tan. Most sunscreens are graded according to a Sun Protection Factor Number system. A good rule of thumb is that the higher the number the more protection it affords. Thus a number 15 product will be suitable for very sensitive skins, while normal skins that are not inclined to burn easily will tolerate a number 6 and olive skins a number 2. Be sure to choose the right SPF number for your skin and don't over-estimate your skin's resilience to sun damage.

4 Protect vulnerable spots

Pay special attention to areas that burn easily, especially the breasts, nose, shoulderblades, backs of knees and feet. Use an extra-strong sunscreen on your face and always smooth a lipscreen over your mouth. Your lips contain no melanin – the pigment granules that rise to the surface of the skin to change its colour and afford protection.

5 Wear a waterproof sunscreen swimming

Ultra-violet burning rays can penetrate below the surface of the sea or a swimming pool so protect yourself with a special waterproof product. After swimming and towelling dry, remember to apply more sunscreen.

The mask of pregnancy

A minority of women develop dark pigmented patches on their skin during pregnancy known as chloasma or 'the mask of pregnancy'. Exposure to the sun makes this condition worse and if you discover that your skin darkens unevenly you should stop sunbathing. It is a nuisance but the affected areas can be concealed easily with special creams and make-up. Buy the products formulated for evening out skin tone, concealing dark rings under eyes and disguising birthmarks. And don't worry – it will disappear eventually but it may be several months after the birth of your child before it fades away altogether. It is caused by the over-stimulation of MSH, a melanocyte-stimulating hormone in the

pituitary gland. It usually appears in the form of brown spots across the nose and cheeks and is more common in brunettes than blondes. A total sunblock or high SPF numbered sunscreen will help protect you when you are outside in the sun. Sometimes birth marks, freckles and moles also darken but staying out of the sun will minimize this, too.

A healthy tan looks attractive and can make you feel good, but you should take special care when sunbathing during pregnancy. Build up your exposure to the sun only very gradually and use a protective sunscreen.

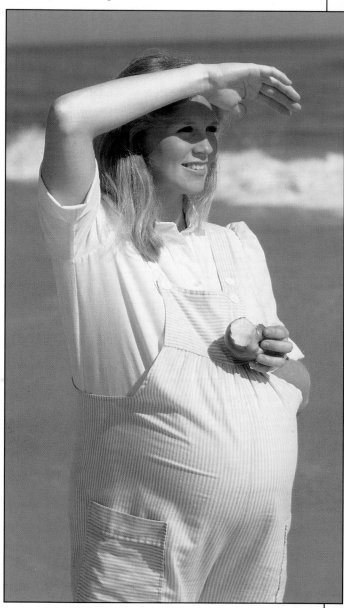

Healthy eating guidelines for pregnancy

If you have been eating along the guidelines laid down for a good diet in the preconceptual period, you have already established a healthy eating pattern. Basically, the best diet is the one that provides all the essential nutrients you need for optimal health. During pregnancy, your requirement for certain nutrients increases as the baby growing inside you makes demands upon you, and your body has to work harder than usual under the added stress.

Many women think that they have to eat large quantities of food and 'eat for two' during pregnancy. They stuff themselves with cakes, biscuits, snack foods and many nutritionally inferior products in the mistaken belief that they are doing the right thing. But although your calorie requirement is higher than usual, it is only marginally so and you need not eat double portions. Yes, you are eating for two but it is the quality of the food you eat, not the quantity that counts.

You need high-quality food for your baby to grow and develop normally and to stay strong, fit and healthy yourself and avoid some of the common pregnancy-related aches and pains. During pregnancy both you and your baby sacrifice nutrients you need for your own bodies if the diet of one of you is inadequate. Thus if you become deficient in a particular vitamin your baby may sacrifice her supply to you. To ensure that this does not happen you must eat a healthy, varied diet which is high in fresh wholefoods and low in processed foods. Your nutritional requirements are higher during pregnancy and lactation than at any other time in your life and if you want an enjoyable pregnancy and a really healthy baby, it is worth making the effort to eat well. No mother wishes to deprive her baby of the nutrients she needs for growth and development.

Scientists and doctors now know that a poor diet which is deficient in essential nutrients can increase the risk of having a stillborn or handicapped baby. Some women who think that they have sufficient to eat and have a healthy diet are malnourished and putting their babies at risk. You must be aware that your baby *is* what you eat to a great extent – she depends on you for an adequate supply of nutrients to meet her needs. In order for you to eat well, you must have a basic knowledge of nutrition and the advantages of eating certain foods. Opposite is a list of which foods you should be eating daily. Just because you have plenty to eat does not mean you are eating the *right* foods.

There are no special dishes or foods that you *must* eat during pregnancy but there are groups of foods that contain important nutrients to fuel your body and build your baby's, which you should eat regularly. And although you may develop cravings for specific foods you must be careful to eat a really varied diet.

You will soon become accustomed to eating the healthy, natural way and will not want or enjoy the low-quality, high-calorie foods you once ate. You will find yourself automatically avoiding sugary, refined and creamy dishes in favour of more wholesome alternatives. And with your new nutritional awareness you will bring your family up to eat along healthier lines and establish good eating patterns for the future.

Your daily food plan

You must eat three nutritious meals a day at regular intervals and not skimp on your food. Pregnancy is *not* the time for controlling or losing weight. You will have to get accustomed to the idea that you will put on some weight but this will quickly disappear after the baby is born, especially if you breastfeed and exercise regularly. However, neither should you gain excessive weight so that you literally balloon. For more advice on sensible weight gain, turn to page 84.

However busy you are, it is important that you should not miss out on meals or go for too long without food. If you work, take a nutritious snack with you to the office or factory – some oatmeal biscuits, fruit, raw vegetables, nuts or cheese. Avoid candy bars, crisps, buns and chocolate – they are all high in unneeded calories and low in goodness.

Look at the chart for a general guide to the helpings of different foods that you should endeavour to eat each day. Of course, it is impossible and would be very boring to lay down exact daily menus for you to follow. This plan is flexible enough for you to choose what you enjoy and vary the dishes throughout the week. Servings

Food	Sources	Quantity
Protein	Meat, fish, poultry, cheese, nuts, beans and pulses, seeds, vegetable proteins etc.	2 servings daily
Eggs	Cooked in any way	3-4 servings weekly
Milk and milk products	Whole, skimmed or semi-skimmed milk, butter-milk, live yoghurt, soft cheeses	4 servings daily
Whole grains and cereals	Wholemeal bread and flour, whole-grain breakfast cereals, eg. granola and muesli, wholemeal rolls and muffins, whole-grain biscuits, brown rice, oatmeal, oatcakes, wheatgerm, bran, wholemeal pancakes etc., buckwheat	4 servings daily
Green leafy vegetables	Cabbage, spinach, lettuce, broccoli, kale, Swiss chard, Brussels sprouts, curly endive, watercress, spring greens etc.	1-2 servings daily
Vitamin C foods	Citrus fruits (orange, grapefruit, tangerine, lime, lemon), green or red peppers, tomatoes, cantaloupe melon, strawberries, blackcurrants, redcurrants, jacket potato	2-3 servings daily: whole vegetables, fruit or squeezed juice
Other fruits and vegetables	Apricots, prunes, plums, peaches, nectarines, dates, cherries, pears, apples, melon, grapes, bananas, berry fruits, corn, salad vegetables, swede, turnip, parsnip, beans, peas, onions, courgettes, carrots, aubergines, cauliflower, pumpkin, leeks, avocado etc.	1-2 servings daily

This chart shows you the number of servings of basic healthy foods that you should try to eat every day. It is very flexible and can be adapted to your personal preferences and to meet the requirements of a busy lifestyle.

are not measured exactly and the amount of food you eat will be conditioned by your appetite and the type of food. For example, four daily helpings of whole-grain cereals may be split in different ways:

1 1 bowl muesli; 1 heaped tablespoon of bran; 1 slice wholemeal bread; 1 helping brown rice.

2 1 bowl granola; 2 slices wholemeal bread; 1 wholemeal pancake filled with savoury mixture.

3 1 wholemeal muffin; 1 slice wholemeal bread; 1 fruit crumble with wholemeal and bran crumble topping; 1 bowl wholewheat cereal e.g. Shredded Wheat.

Use the plan as a framework within which to plan your menus for each day. As a general rule, unless you are vegetarian, you should try to eat liver at least once a week, and drink plenty of mineral water every day.

Typical daily menu

Here is an example of a typical daily menu to help you plan out your meals. In addition to the suggestions given below, you can also enjoy fruit juices, mineral water and herbal tea, and nibble at healthy fresh fruit, nuts and vegetables as the mood dictates. You will never feel hungry although neither will you over-eat. You are guaranteed high-quality

meals every day which are not high in sugar, saturated fats or processed foods laced with additives.

Typical daily menu

Breakfast:
Whole-grain cereal with milk/yoghurt and fresh fruit juice or grapefruit
1 slice wholemeal bread with scraping butter and honey or peanut butter
1 egg, hard-boiled or poached (optional)
Decaffeinated coffee or tea

Mid morning:
Small glass of milk with oatmeal biscuits, dried fruit and nuts

Lunch:
Mixed fresh salad with omelette, quiche or beans or cheese
Slice wholemeal bread
Fruit

Mid-afternoon:
Small carton live yoghurt and/or fresh fruit

Dinner:
Grilled liver, fish, meat, poultry or shellfish or bean/lentil dish
Baked potato with cheese
Green vegetables or salad
Yoghurt and fresh fruit or wholemeal biscuits and cheese or milky dessert

Bedtime:
Hot milky drink (or half milk-half water) or slice wholemeal bread with apple and pear spread or peanut butter

Healthy eating guidelines for pregnancy

You can see that you get plenty to eat and it is all healthy food. It is economical if you wish it to be and need not be expensive. If you are eating on a budget, you can still eat sensibly without spending a fortune. What is expensive is not necessarily the best from a nutritional or flavour point of view. Cheap stewing steak is just as nutritious as fillet steak and makes a delicious casserole, while economical chicken portions or fish fillets are as health-giving as finest Scotch salmon or pheasant and can be served in tasty sauces.

You can make use of cheaper cuts of meat, economical fish and poultry. They are all good sources of protein. Don't forget that cheese, eggs, dried beans, lentils and some vegetables, brown rice and wholewheat pasta also contain protein and many other nutrients. They are all reasonably inexpensive and make interesting meals. Buy seasonal fruit and vegetables when they are cheap and plentiful.

If you have the time and enjoy making things yourself, you will find it is cheaper to make your own bread, live yoghurt, cakes and biscuits than to buy them. They will be more flavoursome and you can control the ingredients you use to ensure that they are of the best quality. You can also be confident in the knowledge that they are free from additives with nothing added or taken away.

Preparing food

You may think that you need read no further and know all about preparing food but how can you be sure that you are handling it correctly? Even the most wholesome ingredients need careful preparation if they are to retain their intrinsic nutritional goodness and flavour. Here are some simple guidelines for you to follow:

1   Always wash or scrub fruit and vegetables thoroughly to remove any traces of chemical sprays and dirt. Peel if necessary.
2   Don't prepare vegetables in advance and leave them soaking for a long time in salted water. They will lose some nutrients.
3   Cut and prepare fruit and vegetables at the last possible moment before eating or cooking. Many start to oxidize and lose their vitamin C content as soon as they are exposed to the air.
4   Always wash oranges and citrus fruit really well if you intend to use the rind in cooking. Some fruit is dyed or waxed to improve its appearance and to make it appear more lustrous.
5   Use only dried fruits that have been sun-dried – not those sprayed with mineral oil to make them more glossy and attractive. The oil can rob you of the essential fat-soluble vitamins, A, D, E and K.
6   Store vegetables in a cool, dark place to protect them against loss of nutrients.
7   If you wish to freeze fruit or vegetables, do so as quickly as possible after picking.
8   When cooking vegetables, steam them for preference. This helps guard against loss of nutrients, especially the water-soluble vitamins B and C which can be partially destroyed by boiling and are lost in the cooking liquid. A steamer is a good investment as the vegetables cook in the steam of the boiling water below without loss of nutrients.
9   If you do boil vegetables, use the minimum of water. Bring it to the boil *before* adding the vegetables and boil hard until tender but still slightly crisp. Do not overcook so that they become mushy. You can use the cooking liquid again for making soups, vegetable stocks and gravies.
10   Never, never add bicarbonate of soda (baking soda) to the cooking water to preserve the bright green colour. It destroys vitamin C as well as giving the food a slightly unpleasant flavour.
11   Always grill, bake or casserole meat rather than frying or roasting it with fat, which adds unnecessary calories and can be a contributory factor in heartburn later on in pregnancy. Speedy cooking methods such as grilling help retain valuable nutrients as well as saving you time.
12   Steam or bake fish in preference to frying for the reasons given above.
13   Make sure that all the food you buy is really fresh – the fresher it is, the higher its nutritional content and the better for you.

The short-cuts to saving time

When you are pregnant or nursing your new baby for that matter, you will not have a lot of time or energy for cooking even though it is essential that

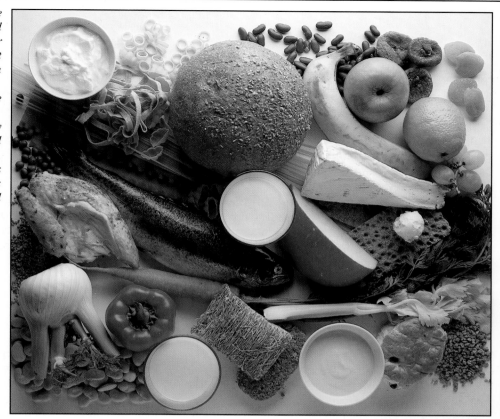

All the foods shown here are nutritious and healthy, and can be included in your pregnancy diet. Fresh fruit and vegetables, whole-grain bread, beans and pulses, dried fruit and nuts, can be combined with fish, poultry, meat, eggs and dairy products to give a varied and appetising food plan. Careful preparation enables you to retain the intrinsic nutritional goodness and flavour of these foods.

you must eat nutritious meals which inevitably involve some preparation. If you don't want to spend hours slaving over a hot stove, you can make use of the range of available modern kitchen gadgets to save time and prepare meals with the minimum of labour. When you are pregnant, a food processor, blender, mixer or freezer becomes a godsend.

Some models are more expensive than others and it is worth shopping around to discover which best suits your budget and your requirements. It is worth investing in a good blender or processor now as it will also be needed for puréeing baby food later on. A processor will take all the effort out of mincing, chopping, slicing, grinding, puréeing soups and vegetables, making cakes and bread, preparing pastry and crumble toppings. It is a very versatile kitchen aid and well worth having.

If you are still at work or kept busy with young pre-school children, then it makes sense to cook in batches and freeze some portions until needed. This is ideal for casseroles, pasta sauces, bread, cakes, stews, pies and flans. They can even be defrosted and reheated in a microwave oven if you are pushed for time. While not essential, a microwave can reduce the cooking time of many dishes drastically

without any loss of flavour. There were doubts raised in the past about the safety of these ovens but any radiation leakage problems seem to have been ironed out and they are now safe to use.

The cooking method you favour is also important and can save time as well as nutrients. For example, grilling is fast but you do need to buy good cuts of meat – tender, lean steak, for example – rather than cheaper, tougher cuts which require longer, slower cooking to tenderize them. You can grill chicken, of course, and fish. Frying is fast but can add unwanted calories and fat, so make sure that you fry foods only in the minimum of oil, not lard or butter which are saturated fats. If you are feeling tired or nauseous, you don't have to cook a big meal – a fresh salad, cheese and whole-grain bread, fruit or yoghurt are all nutritious foods and can make an excellent, quick meal.

It is important that you *enjoy* your food during pregnancy. You should never feel that you are making a sacrifice by cutting out processed convenience meals and eating in a healthier way. In fact, it is to be hoped that you will come to prefer this new diet and make it the pattern for the future. There are lots of recipe suggestions for delicious, nutritious dishes in the coming pages.

Carry on exercising as usual

During the first month of your pregnancy you are probably not even aware of the fact that you have conceived. Most exercise that you do in the first two or three months is unlikely to harm your baby. And the fitter and healthier you are at the time of conception and throughout the duration of your pregnancy, the greater your chances of a healthy baby and a shorter, easier delivery. Many women have run, jogged, cycled, swum and danced their way through pregnancy and they have had the advantages of a greater sense of fitness and physical well-being, less weight gained, a faster recovery after the birth of their babies and a shorter time regaining their figures.

The days have gone where doctors advised pregnant women to stop working and put their feet up for nine months of physical inactivity. Women now know that this led to poor muscle tone, reduced body awareness and, in fact, a body that was ill-prepared for the rigorous demands of labour. Of course, you will need regular periods of rest and relaxation when you are pregnant, but you require exercise, too. So there is no need to stop your sports or active exercise in the first few months unless your doctor advises strongly against it on medical grounds.

As the months pass, you will need to moderate your usual exercise programme as your 'bump' gets larger. In the following pages you will find month-by-month specially adapted antenatal exercises which are suitable at various stages of your pregnancy and take your physical condition and degree of mobility into account. Even during the last month when you may be feeling uncomfortable and less mobile, you can still take positive action to stay fit.

You can either exercise at home or attend the special classes that are now held for pregnant women at many gyms, leisure centres and exercise studios. These usually cater for women from their third month onwards. Work-outs and exercise programmes are devised to build strength and stamina for labour, to maintain muscle tone and flexibility and to teach body awareness. It is

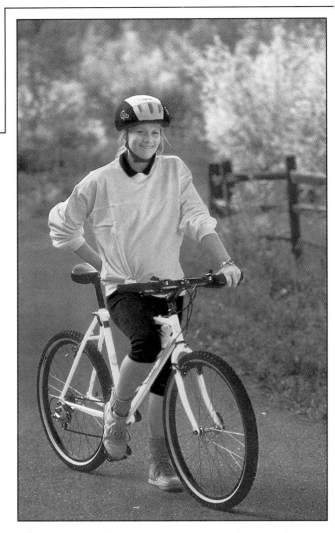

If you enjoy cycling, you can continue doing so for a few more months – or, at least, until your 'bump' grows large. Always be careful not to fall off your bike as any accidents could harm you and your baby.

surprising how little many women know about their own bodies and how they function. During pregnancy you will want to understand more about the internal workings of your body and how they affect the baby growing inside you. An increased awareness of your body acquired through physical exercise can heighten your physical responses and help you to understand your pregnancy better and to be more conscious of your unborn child.

Regular exercise can help teach you to listen to your body, to get to know its limitations and also to realize its potential for endurance and flexibility – two qualities that will be needed in labour. The stronger and more supple your body is, the easier and faster you should be able to give birth to your baby and recover afterwards.

Preconceptual exercise

The best time to start exercising is *before* you get pregnant so that you can build up a level of fitness and strength in advance. This sort of fitness is easier to maintain throughout your pregnancy than if you have to start from scratch in the second or third month. Also, it is important to establish the fitness habit and to make exercise an integral part of your lifestyle and daily routine. If you are used to exercising regularly, it will be less difficult and tiresome to continue doing so throughout your pregnancy.

Someone who is reasonably fit and active before conception can usually continue to swim, cycle, dance, work-out or jog well into their pregnancy as long as she does not feel any discomfort or pain. Inevitably as the months pass and you get heavier, you will find yourself slowing down and you will not be able to achieve what was once possible and normal. Be sure to check with your doctor or midwife if you are worried about exercising during pregnancy.

Why exercise in pregnancy?
1   You will feel fitter, happier and more energetic if you exercise throughout your pregnancy. You will get to know and *like* your body. This is very important as your body assumes new, unfamiliar curves, your waistline thickens, and some fat may build up on upper arms, thighs and hips. Although these may be the inevitable result of hormonal changes within yourself, they can be controlled with regular exercise.
2   Exercise will strengthen your muscles. This is not only important during labour but also in the months leading up to it. During pregnancy your poor muscles have to take a lot of extra strain – for example, if your abdominal muscles are slightly flabby, your lower back muscles will have to bear all the hard work of supporting your spine and this may lead to lower backache – a common enough problem in later pregnancy. Regular exercise can help keep all muscles in good working order – strong and flexible – and thus reduce the risk of backache and other muscular aches and pains.
3   The high pregnancy levels of the hormones oestrogen and progesterone help to soften and relax muscles, so it is more important than ever before to

keep them well-toned and strong. Gentle exercise repeated every day can firm up abdominal, hip and leg muscles and sagging upper arms, and strengthen shoulders, back and chest muscles.
4   As you exercise and tone up these muscles, you will control any extra weight gain in these areas. Although you are not exercising to lose weight, you are toning up the muscles underneath the rounded, fleshy pads that may appear. These trouble-spots will gradually disappear after the baby is born, especially if you breastfeed your child and religiously practise your postnatal exercises.
5   Scientific research has shown that well-toned, strong muscles will help in delivery, too. You can increase your chances of having a shorter, easier labour. Women who are physically fit and exercise regularly throughout their pregnancies suffer fewer complications in labour and 50 per cent less Caesarean births. They have more strength and stamina, are more physically aware of their bodies and how muscle groups work. Thus they are better able to control the contractions and the pace of the birth itself.
6   Aerobic exercise such as walking, cycling, jogging, swimming and dancing promotes cardiovascular fitness – a stronger heart and circulatory system. Thus you can pump oxygen more efficiently to meet the requirements of your baby. Better circulation has beauty spin-offs, too. You are less likely to develop ugly varicose veins in your legs.
7   Cardiovascular fitness can also reduce your chances of suffering many common pregnancy aches and pains – good circulation leads to better bowel action and can prevent constipation and piles.
8   Exercise can help develop stronger back muscles and better posture. You will discover that your weight load shifts forwards as the baby grows and your balance will change as your centre of gravity is situated in your abdomen. You may develop a tendency to throw yourself forwards, or lean backwards to counteract this. Neither is right and will only lead to unnecessary backache. Exercise will strengthen your back and abdominal muscles and help you to walk tall and straight.
9   If you are unused to exercise you may find that it brings a whole new dimension to your life – you will feel more energetic and more confident about your changing body and the whole experiment of being pregnant. You will also have the reassurance of knowing that the more you do to keep yourself in good shape, fit and healthy, the more likely it is that your baby will be healthy, too.

Carry on exercising as usual

10 Last but not least, keeping fit in pregnancy not only speeds up the process of regaining your natural body shape after birth, but it also builds strength and endurance for the task of coping with a small baby and being permanently on call for the first few weeks. This is an emotional time for many women – they feel tired or weak and yet they need to summon up all their reserves of strength to face up to the challenge of caring for a new life. Strong arm and back muscles will help you carry the growing baby in your arms and lift her up from her cot or pram.

If exercise is unfamiliar . . .
If you have not exercised regularly in the past, pregnancy is not the time to embark on a strenuous exercise programme. However, this does not mean that you should continue to be totally inactive. Even if you are very unfit indeed, there is still a wide range of exercises that you can do to improve flexibility, suppleness and muscle tone and strengthen your heart. Do not leave it until the fourth month or even later in your pregnancy. Start now as soon as you discover that you are pregnant.

How do you start? Well, if you are overweight or anxious about your level of fitness you should seek your doctor's advice. Whatever form of exercise you choose, it is important to start off slowly and build up your fitness gradually. The old maxim is: *train don't strain*. This means not trying to run before you can walk and only increasing the number of repetitions of certain exercises, or the distance you swim, walk or cycle as you feel stronger.

Walking is one of the best ways to start exercising. It can be gentle or brisk; you can control the pace and rest whenever you feel tired or breathless. Try to walk for at least 30 minutes every day and make it part of your routine. Although it may not feel particularly demanding or strenuous, walking has cardiovascular benefits and it will help improve your general circulation and increase the oxygen flow to your developing baby. For short shopping expeditions or visiting friends who live locally, walk instead of taking the car. Be sure to wear flat, comfortable shoes with well-cushioned soles as high

heels may distort your natural posture and encourage backache.

If you are tempted to join an exercise class, be sure to tell the instructor that you are pregnant and ask her if there are any exercises that you should not attempt. Concentrate only on gentle exercises with fewer repetitions if you are unfit and out of condition or, better still, join a specially devised antenatal class. Some cater only for women who are more than three months pregnant so you may have to be content with walking, swimming or cycling for a couple of months while you wait.

If exercise is familiar . . .
There is no reason why you should not continue running, walking, cycling, swimming, dancing or working-out throughout your pregnancy if you have achieved a reasonable level of fitness and are used to doing it for at least 20–30 minutes per session three or more times per week. However, if you feel any pain or discomfort you should stop immediately. If pain persists, consult a doctor.

Some fit women continue to jog right through their pregnancies, even on the day that labour starts! Invariably they enjoy easy deliveries, regain their figures quickly and resume running within weeks of the birth. If you are one of them, pay particular attention to your clothing and make sure that it is loose and not restricting in any way. Your shoes should have well-conditioned soles for extra shock absorption as you pound the ground more heavily than usual. Run only on grass. Roads and hard surfaces tend to jar your spine, joints and muscles and may lead to injury. If you have never run before and are reading this, *please* do *not* take up jogging for the first time in pregnancy. Although it is an excellent preparation for pregnancy it may be harmful rather than beneficial if you start training after conception and are unused to the strains it places on your body.

In Month 2's exercise section, there will be a discussion of the different sports and exercises that you can continue to practise during your pregnancy and how to go about it.

Exercise and beauty
Exercise helps increase circulation and thus improves your skin tone and colour. Your facial skin will glow and look healthier, while your body skin should be more elastic, smooth and supple and less likely to suffer from stretch marks in the coming months. Another benefit is that you reduce the risk

of developing cellulite. This is the dimpled looking fat that builds up on hips and thighs and resembles the puckered skin of an orange. During pregnancy the hormonal changes inside you may predispose you to cellulite, and poor circulation and inactivity makes it even more of a certainty. However, regular exercise plays an important role in prevention.

Exercise is just another aspect of beauty and taking care of your body. It will make you feel fitter, better, more confident and attractive. It will also help prevent excessive weight gain so that you can be proud of your body and your new blossoming abdomen – confident in the knowledge that you still look good and that pregnancy can only improve your appearance.

If you do not enjoy cycling, regular brisk walking is good for improving your blood circulation and for increasing the oxygen flow to your developing baby. Gentle jogging (not fast running) can be continued well into your pregnancy, but this is not the time to take up this particular exercise if you are unused to it.

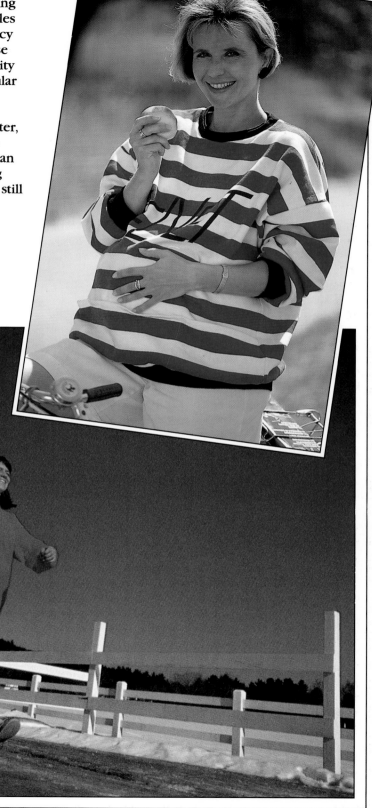

Start enjoying your pregnancy

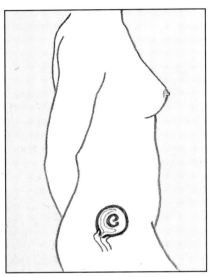

The illustration above shows how at this early stage in your pregnancy the uterus is still relatively small and concealed within the pelvis. Although it will enlarge gradually, you will not see any visible difference until the fourth month. You can see that within just two weeks (between the seventh and ninth weeks) the embryo grows rapidly. Note that these are larger than life size (about 3 times).

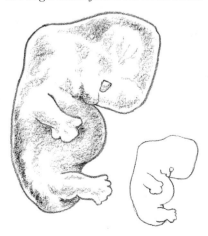

You

By now you will know the truth and your pregnancy will be confirmed. You will be more aware of the changes within your body but your figure and weight will remain the same as always. Your friends may compliment you on your radiance and glowing skin even though you might not have told them yet that you are pregnant. Some women sail through the first trimester (three months) of pregnancy without feeling ill or tired. Others are plagued by fatigue and the dreaded morning sickness. But if you are fit and healthy and eat a good diet, there is no need to feel this way as we shall see. The important thing to bear in mind is that pregnancy is a natural condition – it is not an illness. You do not have to retire from your normal life and put your feet up for nine months or let your partner cocoon you in cotton wool. There is no reason why you should not go on working as usual and lead an active social life for at least seven months as long as you are healthy and strong. Some women even work up to the day they give birth and still feel wonderful. Enjoy your pregnancy and carry on with living – you will find it even more fulfilling that way.

However, even the fittest, healthiest women sometimes suffer ill effects such as moments of dizziness and feeling faint and giddy. Make sure that you eat regular meals, especially a nutritious breakfast. You may find that you go off certain foods or develop a fad or craving for such unlikely things as oysters (if you can afford them) or more everyday foods like chips or oranges – but in the middle of the night! Of course, not every woman experiences this so don't be disappointed if you just eat your normal diet. It is not uncommon to suddenly dislike the taste of alcohol and cigarettes and other unhealthy substances and not want them anyway – perhaps this is your body's way of telling you that they are bad for the baby.

The pregnancy hormones will be hard at work within your body and you will notice changes in your skin and hair. Usually the skin becomes dryer than usual but some women develop an oil problem. Either way you will have to adapt your skin routine accordingly if you have not already done so (*see* pages 16-21). Your hair may be less manageable than usual and will need frequent washing and setting.

Your baby

By the end of the second month your baby is a recognizable human being with a head, trunk, tiny limbs, nostrils, lips, tongue and little webbed fingers and toes. It has the beginnings of a circulatory system and all its major internal organs – liver, kidneys and heart – are developing. Floating in its amniotic sac, its head is a more recognizable shape but still enormous in relation to its tiny body. If you could feel the fetus at this stage it would be soft, but from the eighth week onwards the cartilage that forms its rudimentary skeleton is beginning to change into bone.

Meanwhile, the placenta is starting to form as the lifeline between you and your baby. It transports oxygen and nourishment to the baby and carries away wastes. It grows from a cluster of cells embedded in the uterine wall. Gradually as it starts functioning it controls the production of pregnancy hormones, too. At no time does your blood flow directly into the baby. It can pass only through the tissues on your side of the placenta into the baby on the other side. A membrane separates your bloodstream from that of the baby and the two never mingle. The placenta will not be fully developed until the twelfth week and then it will act as a filter. Everything you eat, drink or even inhale can pass through the placenta into the baby. Not the foods themselves perhaps but substances within them, such as health-giving nutrients as well as the toxins in cigarette smoke, lead from car exhaust fumes or even chemical additives in food. The placenta is not a barrier to harmful substances as was once thought. Therefore you must make an effort to eat and live sensibly if you have not already done so. Inside you, however, your baby is growing fast and is no bigger than a broad bean or your little toe.

Make arrangements now

As soon as your pregnancy is confirmed you will have to start thinking about the sort of birth you want, whether in a hospital or at home. Hospitals vary a great deal in their policy towards birth – some are more enlightened than others which are more technologically-orientated. The choice must be yours. So before you book in somewhere, read as many books as you can about birth and talk to women with different birth experiences so that you can decide whether you want as natural a birth as possible or all the modern facilities and pain-relieving drugs to assist you. Ask your doctor and local representatives of organizations such as LaLeche League and the National Childbirth Trust about the hospitals in your area and which one would be best for you, your medical requirements and attitude to birth.

The embryo floats within an amniotic sac inside the uterus. Already its own life-support system, the placenta, is forming. The embryo itself is still tiny – under 2.5cm/1in long – but it is beginning to move, has arms, legs, a primitive face and ear holes. Weighing less than one ounce, it is recognizable as a miniature human being.

Your beauty plan for nails and hair

2   File the nails to an oval shape with an emery board, filing from each side upwards towards the centre. *Don't* file back and forth.
3   Gently massage in some cuticle cream and then soak for a few minutes in warm soapy water. Remove any dirt with a soft nail brush.
4   Use an orange stick tipped with cotton wool to gently push back the cuticles and remove any dead skin. Dip it in cuticle cream to do this. Dry your

Home manicure

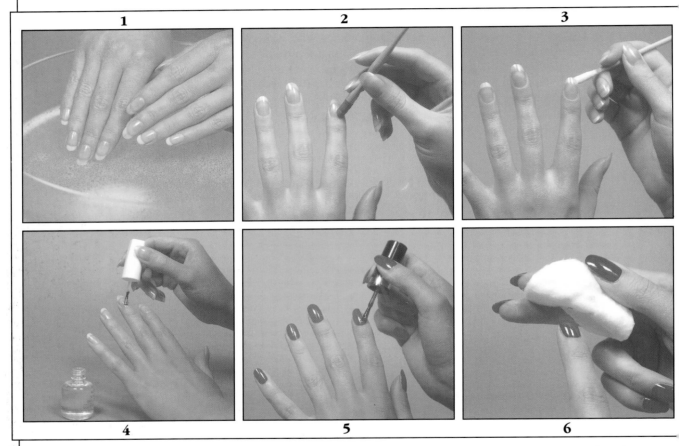

You don't have to visit an expensive salon to enjoy a manicure. You can pamper yourself at home when you are sitting down relaxing one evening. All you need are some nail scissors or clippers, cotton wool balls, a bowl of warm soapy water, emery boards, polish remover, cuticle cream and orange sticks, and some pretty nail polish. You can also use a nail strengthener and a clear varnish for a top coat if wished. A manicure need not take long – under 30 minutes even if you are polishing your nails and waiting for them to dry before applying the top protective coat of clear varnish.
1   Remove any old nail polish with a special oil-based remover using cotton wool pads.

hands and massage plenty of softening hand cream into the skin to moisturize it thoroughly.
5   Now you can apply polish if wished. If your nails are inclined to be brittle, start off by applying a base coat of nail strengthener. When it is dry, apply a coloured polish. Dark polish tends to make nails look longer; pale pearly polishes diminish them.
6   When the polish is thoroughly dry, you may wish to apply another coat. Dry and then apply a protective, hardening, clear top coat to prevent any unsightly chipping which may occur.
Now you should start taking special care of your nails. Just as pregnancy affects the skin in different ways, some women find that their nails become

stronger than ever while a minority complain of brittle, split ones. As a general rule, nails tend to grow faster and stronger during pregnancy, especially if you are eating a healthy diet that supplies plenty of calcium and iron. Taking an iron supplement also tends to make nails healthier. Often, nails are brittle and tend to break easily in the first three months of pregnancy while your body is adjusting to the new stresses imposed on it and then improve in the last two trimesters. If you want to have beautiful hands and nails throughout your pregnancy you should follow these guidelines:

1   Always wear rubber gloves when washing-up and doing household chores such as cleaning, washing and dusting.

2   Wear strong gloves when gardening to protect the hands from dirt, thorns and chemicals.

3   Apply moisturizing hand cream every day, especially after washing your hands which can be drying, and in winter when they may become dry and chafed.

4   Treat yourself to a weekly manicure.

Diet for healthy nails.

Nails should be pink, smooth, strong and flexible – not brittle, ridged and mottled with white spots. They are made of keratin, a form of protein, and their health is directly related to your diet. A doctor can tell a lot about your general state of inner health by examining your nails. The nutrients you need are:

1   **Vitamin A** to help prevent nails splitting and breaking. Liver, cod liver oil, carrots, yellow fruit and vegetables, dried apricots and dark green leafy vegetables will all help promote healthy nails.

2.   **Vitamin B** deficiency çan cause nails to look ridged and to split easily. A daily helping of brewers yeast and yoghurt will help right matters.

3   **Iron** helps make nails look pink and healthy – pale, weak nails may be a result of a lack of this important mineral in your diet. Eat a weekly helping of liver together with eggs, whole-grain cereals and leafy green vegetables. They are best taken with a source of vitamin C for better absorption – oranges, baked potato, tomatoes and peppers, for instance.

4   **Zinc** is rather an overlooked mineral in our food and is often deficient in women who tend to eat an over-refined and processed diet. A tell-tale sign of zinc deficiency is white spots on the nails. A zinc supplement taken with plenty of fresh dark green vegetables, whole-grain cereals, meat and seafood often clears up nail problems.

5   **Calcium** in milk, cheese, eggs, yoghurt and sardines helps keep nails strong and healthy-looking.

6   **Protein** is the main constituent of nails and therefore it is an essential element in your diet, either from animal or vegetable sources.

Eating a healthy diet during pregnancy can often promote rapid nail growth. Take special care of your nails to keep them smooth, strong and flexible. Try regularly manicuring your nails at home to maintain their good condition and to keep them looking attractive.

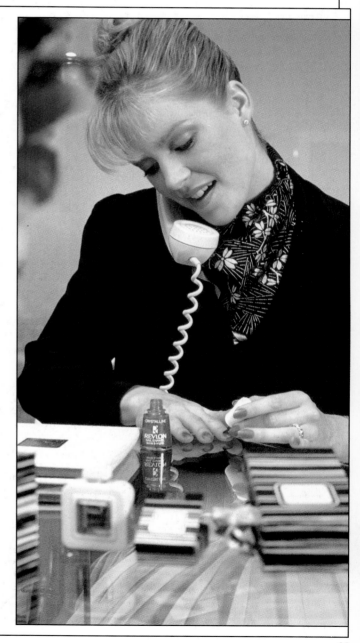

Your beauty plan for nails and hair

Solving nail problems

Most problems encountered with nails can be easily solved by better nailcare and an improvement in diet. Here are some of the common problems that many women experience with hands and nails.

1 **Brittle nails:** apply a protein conditioner and don't polish until the condition improves. Make sure that your diet contains adequate sources of vitamins A and B, protein, calcium and zinc.

2 **Broken nails:** repair with a special, nail-mending kit if they can be saved.

3 **Rough hands:** moisturize regularly and apply a deep-action cream at night to nourish them. If they look red, you can buy a special green-tinted moisturizer to help conceal the redness.

4 **Nicotine stains and age spots:** these are both unsightly, and lemon juice is a good natural treatment. For nicotine stains, wash well and scrub with a nail brush. Dry and rub hard with a cut lemon. Age spots are more difficult to remove, indeed, it may be an impossible task. However, staying out of the sun or protecting your hands with a strong sun-screen will help prevent them getting worse or new liver spots appearing. A once-weekly

treatment with lemon juice and a little oil may also encourage them to fade slightly.

Haircare

Good haircare will help keep your hair in beautiful condition throughout your pregnancy – thick, glossy and soft. Regular shampooing and conditioning combined with careful setting and drying will prevent hair damage and ensure that it is in tip-top condition. You may find that the hormonal changes within your body interfere with the normal condition of your hair. It may improve and become more luxuriant or it may be inclined to break and split and even fall out and get thinner. The important thing is to develop a routine that suits your hair. In order to do this, you must analyze your hair type:

1 Dry hair

This tends to look dull and lack lustre. It is often thin and prone to split ends. Bleaching, colouring and perming may make the condition worse.

Haircare: use a specially formulated shampoo for dry hair and a conditioning rinse. Have a deep conditioning treatment with henna treatment wax or a similar product at least once every three weeks. An occasional oil treatment will protect the hair from moisture loss by coating the cuticles. Just mix about 50ml/2floz oil with the same amount of hot water and massage into your dry hair. Wrap your head in a hot towel to keep in the heat. Leave for 15-20 minutes before shampooing and rinsing really

Analyze your hair type

Hair type	Characteristics	Problems
Normal	Easy to manage, not too dry not too greasy. Washes well and lasts at least 5 days before further washing required. Adapts to most styles.	Encountered only in rare cases when permed or coloured badly
Oily	Lank and dull, prone to dandruff, quickly loses its shape and needs frequent washing with mild shampoo	Dandruff and oiliness, difficult to manage – may be treated by diet as well as by regular shampooing
Dry	Fine, flyaway, lacks gloss and lustre and looks dull. Prone to split ends and needs regular deep-conditioning and cutting	Breaking split ends especially when permed or coloured

You should get to know your hair type and characteristics so that you can deal with any problems you may encounter during pregnancy. The hormonal changes in your body can affect your hair's thickness and strength. Also the food you eat can have an influence on hair condition.

clean in warm water.

The best cream rinses for dry hair usually contains balsam or silicone. Protein treatment packs are also very effective and will restore the hair's strength and flexibility in time. To prevent further damage, never use heated rollers or curling tongs and blow-dry from a safe distance. In the sun, wrap your hair in a scarf or wear a sunhat to prevent dryness.

Causes: these may be unavoidable or a result of neglect and bad haircare routines. Some hair is naturally dry due to a low number of oil glands in the scalp. However, most dry hair is caused by over-colouring, permanent waving, heated rollers, incorrect blow-drying and over-exposure to the sun. Diet may also play an important role. For example, if you are inclined to be anaemic and lack iron, then your hair may be unmanageable, thin, brittle and lacklustre. Taking a course of iron supplements during pregnancy has solved many a dry hair problem. Zinc and sulphur are also essential to keep hair glossy and smooth. Perhaps the most important nutrients of all are the B-complex group of vitamins as deficiencies can lead to dandruff, dryness, lacklustre hair and even premature greying.

2   Oily hair

This usually looks fine the day it is washed but deteriorates rapidly so that by the second or third day it looks and feels greasy.

Haircare: shampoo the hair as often as necessary – every other day or even every day if wished. It will

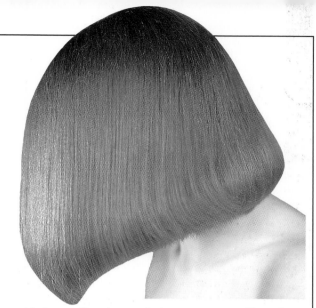

A good haircut will make your hair more manageable and easy to look after in pregnancy.

not make the condition worse. Use a mild shampoo suitable for oily hair. Massage it gently into the scalp and rinse thoroughly. Lemon shampoos are particularly effective as they remove excess oil and leave hair glossy – not dull and lank. Never use a conditioner that contains a lot of oil – it will leave your hair really lank and lacking body. An oil-free conditioner will add body and leave hair feeling silky soft. You can add the juice of one lemon to the rinsing water to help close the follicles and control the oiliness in your hair.

Massage and stimulation of the scalp work wonders for oily hair. Because circulation is often sluggish, it needs stimulation to get adequate oxygen and nutrients. So brush the hair frequently to distribute the oil and make hair shine. Of course, during pregnancy the changes in your hormonal balance may cause oiliness, at least for a short time, so you must know how to treat it.

Causes: oily hair may be a result of large oil glands or an excessive number of them. However, it is often linked to poor diet – one that is rich in fats and over-refined foods. Cutting down on saturated fats, sugar and processed foods and eating a healthy wholefoods diet can often make all the difference to an oil problem.

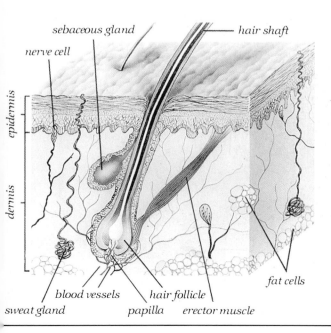

This cross-section through the scalp shows the complex structure of a single hair shaft and the surrounding skin. The growing hair is fed with the nutrients it needs for good condition, health and growth by the network of blood vessels. It receives essential lubricating oils via the sebaceous gland.

sebaceous gland

hair shaft

nerve cell

epidermis

dermis

blood vessels

hair follicle

fat cells

sweat gland

papilla

erector muscle

Your beauty plan for nails and hair

Drying and setting

You probably think that you know how best to dry and set your hair but the method you choose and the way in which you do it may cause damage. Used incorrectly, blow dryers and heated rollers can eventually cause cumulative damage to the outer hair cuticles and even the inner cortex and medulla as well. If you can, it is best to let the hair dry naturally and to handle the hair as little as possible.

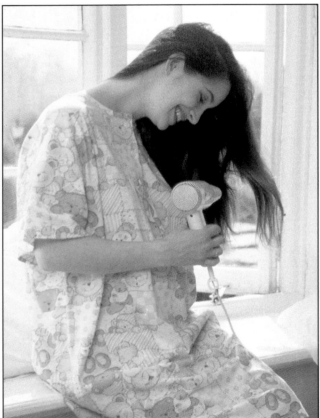

Take care not to damage your hair when drying or setting it. Hair dryers can be very harsh and often lead to dryness and split ends, so hold them well away from your head, or preferably let your hair dry naturally. A heated curling brush will aid easy styling, but should only be used on dry, not wet, hair, to prevent causing damage.

Blow drying

Use a low-wattage dryer and hold it at least 15cm/6in away from your hair, moving it around all the time so that the heat is never concentrated in one spot for too long. Dry your hair in layers to add body and shape – the underneath first, gradually working outwards and upwards. To prevent dryness and split ends, you can spray on a protein-based lotion first to protect your hair from the heat.

Setting

A wet set lasts longer than a dry set using ordinary rollers. You should try to avoid using heated rollers too often however tempting it may be to pop them in first thing in the morning before you leave for work or before a party just to give your hair bounce and fullness. They tend to damage the hair and dry it out leading to brittleness and split ends. To minimize any damage, always wrap some tissue paper round the rollers before winding into your hair. If you insist on using curling tongs which can singe and split hairs, use only on dry, not wet, hair.

Pregnancy hair problems

1   Hair loss: this may be caused by the increased progesterone hormone in your placenta. It may continue after pregnancy but it will grow back again after the birth of your baby – probably thicker than before. The physical stress of pregnancy sometimes causes a minority of the hair follicles to go dormant for a while. When the new hair eventually starts to

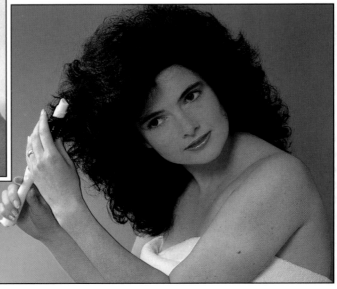

grow and pushes the old hair out you may get what seems to be an unusually large fallout. Also, zinc levels may be low following delivery and a deficiency may be linked with loss of hair until your diet is improved and you get adequate nutrients.

2   Split ends: if your hair becomes very dry, you may have a surfeit of split ends to contend with. Forget everything you ever heard about products

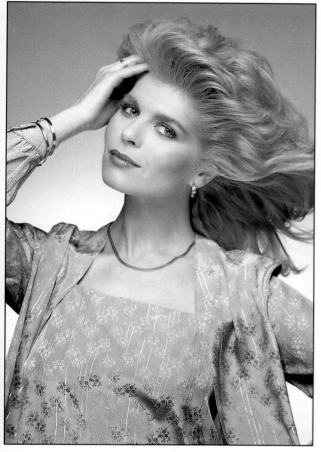

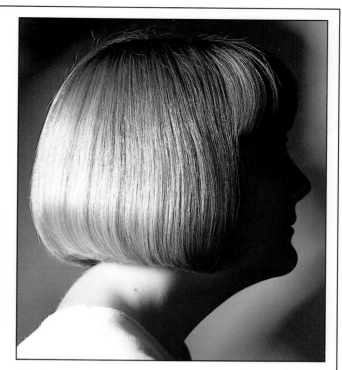

Short hair needs regular cutting to keep it in shape and looking good. On the plus side, however, it requires less attention than longer, full-bodied hair, which needs frequent grooming.

that 'mend' split ends. The best way to get rid of them is to cut them off and then use a moisturizing conditioner as outlined in the section on dry hair (see page 34). Be careful not to hold the dryer too close to your head or use too hot a setting, and steer clear of heated rollers and curling tongs. To avoid split ends, use a bristle brush, protect the hair from the sun and heat and avoid perms and harsh colourants.

3   Perming: even if you normally perm your hair, you may be well advised not to do so during pregnancy while your hormones are somewhat

erratic. It is impossible to know how your hair will react to a perm at this time. Although it will probably be OK, there is a possibility that it may fall out, go frizzy or just not take. Try a different style instead – ask your hairdresser for advice and look through the glossy magazines for ideas. A layered look instead of a perm may add body and fullness to your hair. The next time to have a perm is three to six months after the birth of your baby when your hormones are settling down again.

4   Hairstyles: most women don't want a fussy style that requires a lot of care and time spent on it when they are pregnant, especially in the last trimester when they are starting to feel uncomfortably heavy, and hairwashing and drying are a tiresome chore. An easily manageable style is a good idea – a fashionably short cut or layered look which can be quickly shampooed and finger-dried suits many women. If you like to wear your hair long, keep it simple. You can always ring the changes by pinning it up or pulling it back off the face with pretty combs and clips. Don't use rubber bands, though, especially if you already have dry hair as they will exacerbate the damage and cause split ends.

Get back to food basics and salad freshness

There some essential foods that you must try to eat every day when you are pregnant. You can either buy them or make them yourself – it all depends on how much time you have and whether you enjoy cooking. As we said before, it is important that you try to use really high-quality, fresh and nutritious ingredients – most of which are now available from supermarkets and corner shops as well as health food stores.

Wholemeal bread – the staff of new life

Bread made with 100 per cent wholemeal flour is more nutritious and higher in fibre than white bread. If you aren't accustomed to eating it, you should try to get hooked on it now that you are pregnant. When you buy a loaf, ask the sales assistant or check the label to ensure that there are no unnecessary additives such as artificial colouring, caramel and preservatives. When you find a source that sells delicious bread made with 100 per cent wholemeal flour, you could buy several loaves or rolls at a time and freeze some for later use.

However, you may decide to make your own bread. It is quite easy, especially if you have a food processor with a plastic dough blade to take the hard work out of kneading. This recipe will make one large or two small loaves:

Quick processor wholemeal bread

550g/1lb 4oz/5 cups 100 per cent wholemeal flour
10ml/2 level teaspoons sea salt
1 packet easy blend dried yeast, eg. Harvest Gold
30ml/2 tablespoons sunflower oil
300ml/½ pint/1¼ cups water at blood heat
30ml/2 tablespoons molasses
Optional:
60ml/4 tablespoons cracked wheat
100g/4oz/1 cup chopped walnuts

Using the plastic dough blade, mix the flour, salt and yeast in the food processor quickly. With the machine operating, pour the oil, water and molasses through the feed tube and process for about 1 minute until you have a smooth, elastic dough that leaves the sides of the bowl clean. Shape into a round, place in an oiled bowl and tie up in a plastic bag. Leave in a warm place for about 1 hour until well-risen and more or less doubled in size. Turn out onto a lightly floured board and knock back to get rid of any air. Mix in the chopped nuts or cracked wheat if used and knead lightly. Shape into one large or two small loaves and place in greased loaf tins. Cover with a cloth and leave in a warm place for 30 minutes to 'prove' – until the dough rises to the top of the tin(s). Glaze the top with salt water, milk or egg and bake in a hot preheated oven at 230°C, 450°F, gas mark 8 for 25–30 minutes. Cool on a wire tray. Makes 1 large or 2 small loaves.

Yoghurt for health

Yoghurt is one of the most useful and nutritious foods you can eat now. It is very versatile and is the perfect dessert mixed with fresh fruit; delicious as a topping for muesli or breakfast cereal; great in salad dressings; and a good low-calorie snack. Although practically every food store now sells yoghurt, you should buy the 'live' sort for preference. Most of the yoghurts on the supermarket shelves have been

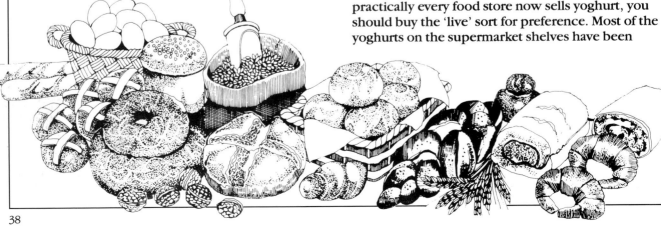

pasteurized *after* the culture is added to prolong their shelf life, but this destroys the beneficial lactobacillus bacteria that helps keep your intestines healthy and manufacture B vitamins there.

Another good reason for purchasing 'live' yoghurts in health food stores and delicatessens or making your own is that many commercial brands contain white sugar, preservatives, artificial colourings and flavourings. Fortunately, some manufacturers are now displaying a trend towards yoghurt which is flavoured with fresh fruit only and contains no additives or sugar.

Home-made yoghurt tastes delicious and is very economical when the cost is compared to buying the equivalent amount in the shops. A special yoghurt-maker is inexpensive and a good investment if you are a yoghurt addict and plan to make it every week. Otherwise, you can use a wide-necked thermos flask or insulated jar. When making yoghurt it is essential to insulate it at a steady temperature during the incubation period as the bacteria are destroyed at temperatures over 48°C, 120°F, and inactive below 32°C, 90°F. Always boil the milk first (cow's or goat's) to avoid any bacteria in the milk fighting the yoghurt bacteria.

Home-made yoghurt

550ml/1 pint/2½ cups milk
15ml/1 tablespoon skimmed milk powder
30ml/2 tablespoons natural 'live' yoghurt

Mix the milk and skimmed milk powder and heat until boiling. Remove from the heat and cool to 43°C, 110°F. Use a sugar thermometer for an accurate reading. Stir the natural yoghurt into the warm milk and pour into a *warmed* wide-necked thermos flask or insulated jar. Seal and leave for a minimum of 6 hours. However, do not incubate for too long or the yoghurt will taste very sour. It should be pleasantly tart. When the yoghurt is of a thick, custard-like consistency, transfer it to a clean container and refrigerate for about 24 hours before serving. Eat on its own or with flavourings of your choice. Makes 550ml/1 pint/2½ cups.

Note: the addition of the skimmed milk powder makes the yoghurt thicker and creamier. Good flavourings for yoghurt are chopped fresh fruit, chopped nuts, muesli or granola, seeds, bran, wheatgerm, honey and spices.

Eat a salad every day

You should try to eat one raw salad meal every day. Salads are among the healthiest food you can eat – high in vitamins and minerals and low in calories. Add protein by using cooked wholewheat pasta, brown rice, beans, nuts, fish, meat, chicken, boiled eggs, cheese or even a yoghurt salad dressing. If your salads tend to consist of some wilting lettuce, limp tomato slices and a piece of dried up beetroot or cucumber, then think again. You *can* be adventurous with salads and make them interesting and varied no matter what the time of year. Here are some ideas for fresh ingredients that you can use either in summer or in winter:

Summer: Lettuce, watercress, curly endive, spinach leaves, sorrel, fennel, tomatoes, garden peas, tender young broad beans, beetroot, raw courgettes and mushrooms, cucumber, spring onions, radishes, red and green bell peppers, nectarines, grapefruit, redcurrants, apricots, almonds, hazelnuts, walnuts, seeds and sprouted grains, mung and alfalfa sprouts.
Winter: Chinese leaves, shredded red or white cabbage, grated carrot, celery, sliced onion, chicory, radicchio, watercress, celery, mushrooms, raw cauliflower florets, red and green peppers, grapes, oranges, apples, pears, lychees, tangerines, bananas, pineapple, almonds, walnuts, hazelnuts, Brazils, pine nuts, seeds and sprouts.

Here are a few quick salads for you to try. They are all simple to make and taste wonderful.

Spinach and blue cheese salad

450g/1lb young spinach leaves
100g/4oz sliced button mushrooms
4 rashers streaky bacon, crisply grilled
75g/3oz blue cheese, cubed
45ml/3 tablespoons olive oil
juice of 1 lemon
dash wine vinegar
1 hard-boiled egg, sliced or chopped

Wash the spinach carefully and discard any tough stalks and damaged leaves. Mix with the mushrooms and crumble the bacon on top. Add the cheese and toss in the oil, lemon and vinegar dressing. For extra protein, add some sliced or chopped hard-boiled egg if wished. Makes 2-3 servings.

Get back to food basics and salad freshness

Pasta and vegetables in parmesan dressing

450g/1lb pasta spirals or other shapes
225g/8oz assorted vegetables such as:
courgettes/zucchini, cut in rounds or matchsticks
broccoli, trimmed into very small flowerets
mange-tout/pea pods, ends trimmed
carrots, cut in rounds or matchsticks
celery, cut in matchsticks
cucumber, cut in matchsticks
spring/green onions, thinly shredded or sliced
asparagus tips
French/green beans, sliced
red or yellow peppers, thinly sliced
Dressing:
140ml/¼ pint/½ cup olive oil
45ml/3 tablespoons lemon juice
15ml/1 tablespoon sherry pepper sauce

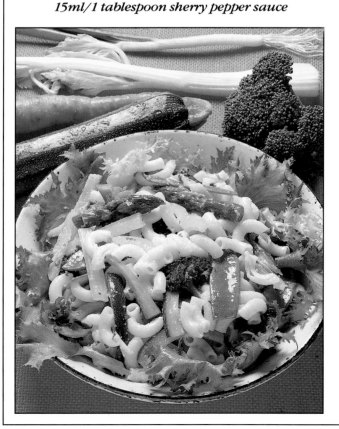

15ml/1 tablespoon chopped parsley
15ml/1 tablespoon chopped basil
60g/2oz/¼ cup freshly grated Parmesan cheese
30ml/2 tablespoons mild mustard
salt and pepper

Cook pasta in a large saucepan of boiling salted water with 15ml/1 tablespoon oil for 10-12 minutes or until just tender. Rinse under hot water to remove starch. Leave in cold water. Place all the vegetables except the cucumber into boiling salted water for 3 minutes until just tender. Rinse in cold water and leave to drain. Mix the dressing ingredients together. Drain the pasta thoroughly and toss with the dressing. Add the vegetables and toss to coat. Refrigerate for up to 1 hour before serving. Serves 6.

Salmon salad dip

225g/8oz can red or pink salmon
225g/8oz/1⅓ cups cottage cheese with chives
15ml/1 tablespoon tomato ketchup
10ml/2 teaspoons Worcestershire sauce
15ml/1 tablespoon chopped parsley

Blend all the ingredients together. Season with salt and pepper to taste. Place in a small dish on a plate and surround with fresh vegetable crudités: for example, carrot, cucumber, cauliflower, celery, red and green peppers, and mushrooms. Sprinkle the dip with chopped parsley before serving.

Lentil tomato salad

175g/6oz brown Continental lentils
1 small onion, chopped
2 spring onions/scallions, chopped
3 tomatoes, quartered
60ml/4 tablespoons olive oil
15ml/1 tablespoon lemon juice or wine vinegar
chopped parsley and mint
1 hard-boiled egg, sliced

Wash the lentils, then cover with water and cook for about 1¼ hours or until tender. Drain and mix with

Try to eat salads every day as they are high in vitamins and minerals and low in calories. Pasta and vegetables in Parmesan dressing (left) is a filling and tasty recipe.

the onion and tomato. Toss in the olive oil and lemon/vinegar. Season and sprinkle with plenty of chopped fresh parsley and mint. Serve with sliced hard-boiled eggs. Makes 3 servings.

Waldorf salad

4 sticks celery, diced
4 apples, red-skinned and green-skinned, diced
180g/6oz grapes, black and white, halved and seeded
120g/4oz/1 cup walnuts or pecans, roughly chopped
300ml/½ pint/1 cup prepared mayonnaise
60ml/4 tablespoons double cream
juice of half a lemon

Mix the celery, apples, grapes and nuts together and toss with the lemon juice. Lightly whip the cream, fold into the mayonnaise. Fold the dressing into the salad and serve chilled. If desired, substitute raisins for the grapes and garnish with 30ml/2 tablespoons chopped parsley. Serves 6.

Hot chicken and spinach salad

175g/6oz young fresh spinach leaves, washed and shaken
6 small spring onions, trimmed
30ml/2 tablespoons flaked hazelnuts
3 courgettes, sliced very thinly
2 boned and skinned chicken breasts
120ml/8 tablespoons olive oil
1 small onion, finely chopped
1 clove garlic, crushed
30ml/2 tablespoons white wine vinegar
salt and freshly ground black pepper
15ml/1 tablespoon chopped fresh tarragon
1 small red pepper, seeded and finely chopped

Tear the spinach leaves into pieces and mix them in a bowl with the spring onions, hazelnuts and courgettes. Cut the chicken into very thin strips. Heat 90ml/6 tablespoons olive oil in a large shallow pan. Add the chicken strips, onion and garlic and fry briskly until the chicken is just tender. Stir in the remaining olive oil, vinegar and seasoning to taste. Add the tarragon and allow to bubble for one minute. Spoon the hot chicken and dressing over the salad ingredients in the bowl and toss together. Sprinkle with the chopped red pepper and serve.

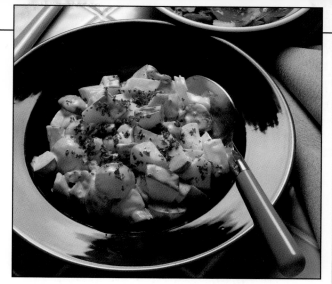

Waldorf salad makes a colourful dish to be eaten on its own as a light meal or as a side dish to accompany a main course.

Oriental salad

1 cake tofu, cut into small cubes
140ml/¼ pint/½ cup vegetable oil
120g/4oz mange-tout/pea pods, ends trimmed
60g/2oz mushrooms, sliced
60g/2oz broccoli flowerets
2 carrots, peeled and thinly sliced
4 spring/green onions thinly sliced
2 sticks celery, thinly sliced
60g/2oz/½ cup unsalted roasted peanuts
120g/4oz bean sprouts
½ head Chinese leaves/cabbage, shredded
Dressing:
45ml/3 tablespoons lemon juice
10ml/2 teaspoons honey
5ml/1 teaspoon grated ginger
45ml/3 tablespoons soy sauce
dash sesame oil

Drain tofu well and press gently to remove excess moisture. Cut into 1.25cm/½ inch cubes. Heat 30ml/2 tablespoons from the 140ml/¼ pint/½ cup oil in the wok or frying pan. Save the remaining oil for the dressing. Cook the mange-tout/pea pods, mushrooms, broccoli, carrots and celery for 2 minutes. Remove the vegetables and set them aside to cool. When cool mix them together with the onions, peanuts and bean sprouts. Mix the dressing and pour over the vegetables. Add the tofu and toss carefully. Arrange a bed of Chinese leaves/cabbage on a serving dish and pile the salad ingredients on top to serve. Serves 4.

Keep fit with your favourite sport

During the second month of pregnancy you can still continue to do most exercises and participate in your usual sports. You may not feel very pregnant yet – your 'bump' is still non-existent and you look the same as usual. However, momentous changes are taking place within your body already and you should not push yourself beyond your usual limits. Just continue exercising in a sensible way without any strain or excessive exertion.

As mentioned before, you can continue jogging, swimming, working-out and dancing. They are all good aerobic exercises. Cycling and riding are OK in the early months but you must be even more vigilant and safety conscious than usual, especially on busy roads. A fall could damage you and your baby. Just take it easy and don't take unnecessary risks. So what are the sports and forms of exercise that you can pursue and how should you go about them?

Swimming

This is probably the best form of exercise during pregnancy. Not only does it strengthen your cardiovascular system and increase blood circulation but it also tones muscles and keeps your figure firm and streamlined. And all this in a state of near weightlessness supported by the water and without putting unnecessary strain on your uterus and abdominal muscles.

You can really enjoy swimming as your body weight increases. The warm water of an indoor pool will help support you and it is very soothing and relaxing, particularly in the last months when you are feeling heavy and uncomfortable. Then it is bliss to sink into the warm blue water of a pool and feel physical encumbrances slip away for half an hour. Most women live within easy walking or driving distance of an indoor swimming pool. Try to visit it two or three times a week as swimming is therapeutic and very beneficial. The resistance of the water against your body will give you a good work-out and exercise and strengthen most muscle groups.

Try not to feel self-conscious about your expanding figure when you strip down to your swimsuit and slide into the water. You can be proud of your new curves. The best way to overcome these feelings is probably to go swimming with your family or a friend who will not pass comment, and to attend the pool at a quiet time of day when there are few spectators present. The pool will be less full, too, and the likelihood of being leapt on by enthusiastic small boys is significantly reduced.

Remember your breathing when you swim – slowly and rhythmically – and take it easy. You are not training for a competition – just trying to stay fit and healthy and enjoying a quiet swim. It is always a good idea to practise a few gentle warm-up exercises (see pages 72 and 73) before you swim and to relax and cool down afterwards before showering and dressing. The golden rules are: don't swim in cold water and don't dive or belly-flop into the pool.

Working-out and dancing

Even if you are used to working-out in a gym or at home by yourself several times a week or attending regular dance classes, you should take special care during pregnancy, particularly after the third month. It might be a good idea to transfer if possible to a pregnancy-related work-out class and to work-out under the supervision of a trained instructor with experience in this field. However, if this is not possible, you should become more discriminating in your choice of exercises and the number of repetitions you perform. Cut out any strenuous sit-ups and other exercises that put excessive strain on the abdominal, back and uterus muscles. Also, any exercises not in the pregnancy work-out that require you to lie on your back while you perform them as the pressure of the uterus may affect the large blood vessels in your pelvis and interfere with normal circulation and blood flow to your baby.

If there are no special antenatal exercise classes in your area, you can follow the step-by-step exercises photographed in this book and devise your own work-out, safe in the knowledge that they cannot harm your baby. The main thing to remember is never to over-strain yourself and to warm-up first to stimulate blood flow to muscles and tissues, loosen tight muscles and joints, and prevent injuries.

Always wear loose clothing in which you feel comfortable. It may be a stretchy leotard and maternity tights, a soft track suit, a baggy T-shirt and warm tights, or loose-fitting trousers to keep the leg muscles warm and prevent cramping. Although synthetic fibres are very elastic and stretch with you, you may find that natural fibres like cotton are better as they allow your body to breathe more easily and absorb perspiration from the skin. As some of the exercises will be performed on the floor or standing in the same spot you need not wear shoes. Avoid any vigorous jogging on the spot, jumping jacks and other fast-moving aerobic exercises.

If you work-out at home, you can buy a special pregnancy exercise tape or video to inspire you and set the right pace and rhythm. Or you can study the exercises in this book and put on a favourite tape or record with a good beat – not too fast, not too slow. Exercise on a thick carpet or mat – it will make any groundwork easier. It's cold and painful working-out on a hard floor.

Some points to remember when you are exercising during pregnancy:

1   Study the exercises and practise the postures and movements before you work-out so that you are familiar with them all. Gradually build them up into a routine so that you can perform them instinctively, effortlessly and without reference to a book.

2   Although I have introduced new exercises each month throughout the book, it is your body and muscle tone that decides which you can do at a particular stage in your pregnancy. Be flexible about your choice of exercise.

3   Some days you may feel more tired than usual and not want to exercise. That's OK. Your body is telling you that it needs a rest, so practise some conscious relaxation techniques instead (see page 144). However, on other days you may feel extremely energetic and tempted to push yourself beyond your usual quota of exercise. Do not overdo it and pay the price with fatigue and aching muscles the following day.

4   Be sure to breathe properly while you exercise – deeply and slowly so that you have sufficient oxygen to fuel your muscles and supply your baby. Do not pant or allow yourself to become short of breath. Stop and relax immediately if you feel breathless.

Cycling

This is another aerobic form of exercise that is good for your heart and lungs and circulatory system. Cycling tones up muscles you did not know you had in your legs and is a great all-round conditioner. Because it improves circulation in the legs without putting too much weight on them, it helps guard against varicose veins, too. If you are a good cyclist with an innate sense of balance, there is no reason why you should not cycle throughout your pregnancy. However, as your abdomen grows larger

your centre of gravity will shift and you may find that this affects your sense of balance. Leaning forwards over the handlebars can ease out your back in later pregnancy but may make arms and shoulders ache so make sure that you can reach the pedals and handlebars comfortably.

Weigh up the pros and cons of continuing to use your bike. Safety is particularly important as a fall could damage your baby as well as you, and you may decide that cycling is not worth the risk and you would be better off switching to another form of exercise until after the baby is born. You must watch out for potholes and uneven road surfaces and take special care when cycling in traffic. Do not cycle up steep hills and put unnecessary strain on your body. Make sure that your bike is in good working order and that the brakes are effective. If you plan to cycle at night, you must have lights on your bike and should wear some white clothing or a fluorescent jacket, armband or reflective strip so that motorists can see you in their headlights.

Most women find that although cycling is OK in early pregnancy, it becomes progressively difficult and more risky in the later months and they turn to some other form of transport or exercise.

Horse riding

The same goes for horse riding. If you have a horse or ride regularly you may wish to continue throughout your pregnancy. However, it is a potentially dangerous sport and it is not worth the risk of taking a tumble when you are pregnant. Get someone else to exercise your horse and resume your riding after the birth when you are fully recovered.

Running and jogging

Although you can jog your way to motherhood, these activities are for the experienced and very fit only and should not be attempted in pregnancy by anyone how has not jogged previously. Like other sports, you should ask your doctor's advice on whether to continue running. Run at a gentle even pace on grass to avoid jarring your joints and spine. Pay special attention to your shoes and ensure that they are well-cushioned as your feet pound the ground many hundreds of times per mile!

Use your warm-up exercises to prepare yourself for running and to cool down and recover afterwards. In later months, you may find that a combination of walking and running is best. As the walking takes over from the running and you grow

Keep fit with your favourite sport

During pregnancy, walking is one of the most enjoyable and beneficial forms of exercise that you can do. Walk briskly, breathe deeply and enjoy the scenery.

heavier, it is a good idea to stop running altogether and wait until your body is getting back to normal again after the birth of your baby before restarting.

Yoga

For many women this is the perfect form exercise for pregnancy. Not only does it work-out and stretch your muscles but it also helps you understand better the way your body works and to be more aware of your breathing. Both these factors are invaluable in labour, and many devotees claim that it helps them to approach childbirth with the right attitude of mind and to cope better with their pregnancies. Yoga can reduce stress and tension and make you feel more contented and relaxed within yourself. It stresses the importance of breathing which, of course, is invaluable in labour when you seek to control the contractions and the pain through a combination of controlled deep breathing and panting.

There are two principles at the heart of yoga: meditation, and the basic *asanas*, or postures. The *asanas* are designed to exercise different areas of your body in slow, controlled movements. If practised regularly, they will help make you more supple and flexible, and strengthen your muscles. Most yoga poses are suitable when you are pregnant and some, such as the 'angry cat', are positively beneficial in relieving backache and other pregnancy pains. Yoga is also helpful in exercising the pelvic region in preparation for childbirth.

Your posture will improve also if you practise yoga, making you feel more comfortable and allowing your baby more room to grow and stretch out inside you. The other aspect of yoga that goes hand-in-hand with the *asanas* is meditation, for the mind and body are inter-related and should always be in perfect harmony giving you a feeling of inner calm and well-being that can be transmitted to your baby. As you practise and master the *asanas* you will develop better control and awareness of your body as well as a new sense of inner peace. Your mind will be free to meditate and you will be more tranquil.

If you would like to take up yoga in pregnancy,

find out if there are any classes in your area. Tell the instructor that you are pregnant and ask advice on how to start and which exercises are safe for you to practise in your condition. You and your baby will find it is a gentle and beneficial way to exercise.

Other sports

Many women play golf throughout their pregnancies. It is relatively gentle compared to most active sports and involves some healthy walking. During the later months, swinging the club may put too much stress on your body, especially your back, as you twist round. If so, refine your game and be content with walking the course and some gentle putting.

If you play tennis and badminton regularly, you may have to give up after the fourth month or so and switch to a less jerky form of exercise where speed and agility are not essential.

Do not snow-ski, water-ski, or lift heavy weights. They are all dangerous activities during pregnancy. Whereas skiing may lead to a nasty fall, even weight-training with light weights can put undue strain on your abdominal and back muscles. You can always resume these sports *after* pregnancy.

In general, whatever sport or exercise you practise, you should aim for gentle, smooth movement and avoid bursts of acceleration, fast changes in direction and body turns, and excessive bouncing up and down. If you have any doubts at all about exercise, do consult your doctor and ensure that there are no medical objections. Be prepared for the fact that some doctors are still of the old school and believe that pregnancy is a time for rest and relaxation and not for exercise. However, if you have a specific medical condition that prevents you exercising and necessitates rest, do take advice and do not risk harming your baby.

Otherwise feel free to exercise as usual, or with sensible modifications so that you do not over-strain yourself. If you follow the month-by-month advice in this book, you will be able to gradually change the type of exercises performed and their frequency and intensity as your pregnancy progresses. However, do remember that walking is essential and you should try to walk somewhere every day – to a friend's house, to work, to the shops or the library. You do

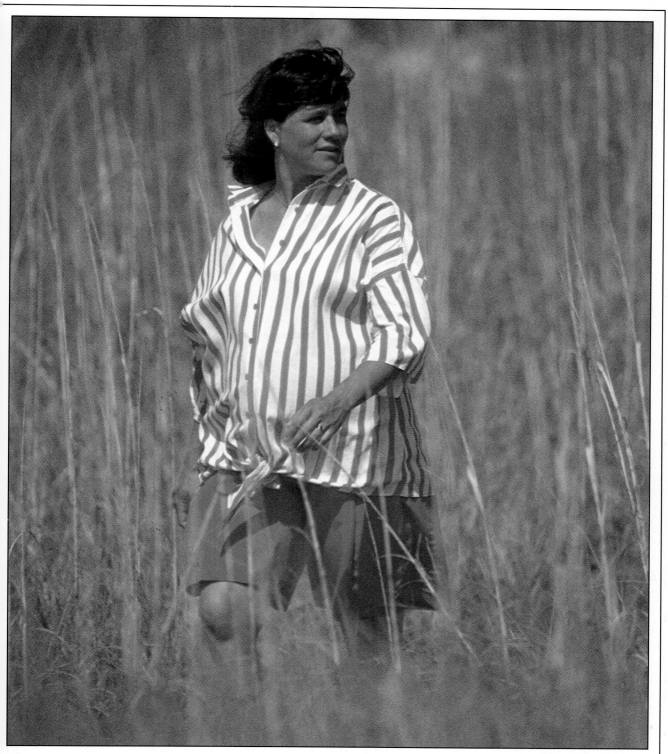

not need an excuse to walk – why not go for a walk because you enjoy it and because you know that it is a great aerobic exercise and is doing you good. It is exhilarating and surprisingly soothing to go out walking on a fine day. You may discover your locality and interesting landmarks or breathtaking views that you never noticed before. It may be more fun if you walk with your partner or a friend.

Look after your health and beauty

You

By the end of the first trimester you will feel much better. You will have adjusted physically and psychologically to the experience of being pregnant. You will be feeling less tired and more in tune with your body and the momentous changes taking place inside you. If you had sickness in the early weeks it should be wearing off by now and although you probably do not *look* pregnant to the rest of the world, you are beginning to *feel* it. You will start to put on weight now – almost imperceptibly at first. You may find, however, that clothes that once fitted comfortably already feel a tiny bit tight. There is no visible 'bump' as yet but at around the twelfth week your womb starts to rise out of the pelvis.

Meanwhile, there will be other visible changes. The skin around your nipples will be getting darker. These marked differences in your skin tone and colouring are caused by the production of pregnancy hormones inside you. Your skin may also start to feel dryish and tight. Using a good moisturizing body lotion after bathing will help counteract any dryness. Alternatively, you can add a few drops of bath oil to the water – choose a luxurious, beautifully scented oil to make you feel really good. One benefit you will receive from now on is that if you have any tell-tale wrinkles and lines on your face, they may appear softer and less obvious than before: a definite plus for any woman.

Now is the best time to visit the dentist for a check-up as your gums may be softening and dental hygiene is more important than ever. Not only are you more likely to get a gum infection now but your teeth are more inclined to fall out during pregnancy than at any other period in your life. Eating a healthy diet and regular brushing (at least twice a day first thing in the morning and last thing at night) will be helpful.

Many women at this time worry about their pregnancy and have mixed feelings about what is to come, even if the baby was planned and looked forward to. If you feel like this, don't worry because it is quite normal. A new baby is a great responsibility and will inevitably bring about changes in your life and your usual routine but you will discover that it is well worth it. A baby is a source of great joy for you and your partner. If you feel nervous, anxious or on edge, try to talk about your feelings to your partner and explain how you feel. It may also help to talk to some girlfriends, especially those with babies or young children of their own. They have been through it all and can offer moral support and advice. Of course, not all women feel like this. Some are lucky enough to avoid the perils of sickness, tiredness and depression and have never felt better in their lives. You may well be one of these, especially if you look after yourself and follow the advice on eating and relaxing.

Regular exercise also helps to keep you feeling good – it is still too early to practise special antenatal exercises only and you can carry on with your usual fitness regime – whether it's running, swimming, walking briskly,

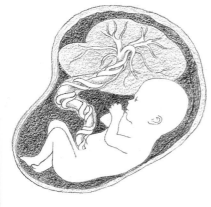

By the end of the third month the placenta is starting to function, supplying the baby with nourishment and excreting waste products. It acts rather like a filter, as blood passes through the tissues on your side and the baby's blood passes through on her side. At no time do the two bloodstreams mix.

cycling, weight-training or working-out. Just be careful that you do not over-strain yourself or get too tired. Exercise is supposed to make you feel better and more energetic – not wear you out.

Your baby

By the time you are 12 weeks pregnant your baby will have her basic organs and limbs. She has nearly completed the early phase of her development and now she can get on with growing in readiness for her entry into the outside world. By the end of the third month she will have finger and toenails, eyelids and a fully functioning placenta.

Blood circulates through the cord and deoxygenated blood is pumped out by the heart back to the placenta together with waste products for excretion. Nutrients from the food you eat enter the baby in the same way to feed her rapidly growing cells. At no time do the cells in your blood mix with those of your baby in the placenta although they do come into close contact. Your respective bloodstreams are separated by a membrane through which nutrients and protective antibodies can be diffused.

The placenta is your baby's lifeline – her only contact with the outside world. Thus it is essential to keep it healthy, strong and functioning normally. It is the vehicle for all the goodness your baby needs to grow and flourish. When you eat a healthy, nutritious diet, the placenta will grow large and produce a range of hormones, notably oestrogen and progesterone, which control the changes in your body during pregnancy.

At the end of the third month your baby, now known as a fetus, is about 10cm/4in long. Although she is still very small, she can suck strongly, frown, clench her fists and press her lips together. Of course, you cannot feel her doing these things, but you may be aware of her kicking you by the end of the next month. Already she has a recognizable face with the chin, tiny snub nose and large forehead that are typical of every young baby.

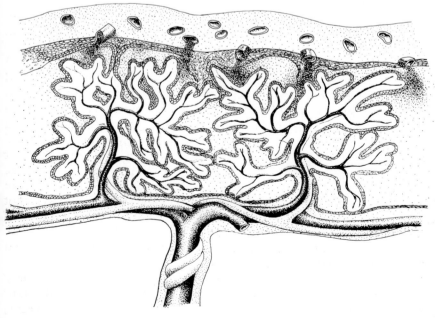

This cross-section through the placenta shows the maternal arteries and veins and the umbilical cord. Your blood filters through the intervillous spaces. Nutrients can slip through and be transferred to the baby. In the same way, waste products can be transferred to the mother. Do remember that other harmful substances can also percolate through this sieve, including drugs and toxic chemicals.

Stay fresh and be a bathing beauty

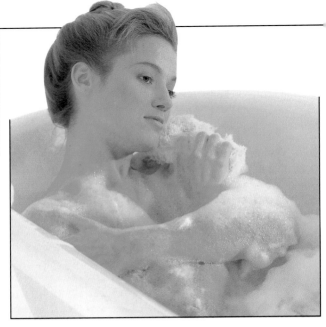

When you are pregnant, a long, luxurious bath is very restful and a good occasion for pampering yourself. At the end of a busy tiring day, a soothing bath can ease away fatigue and help induce a restful night's sleep. This is very important during the first trimester when you will probably feel more tired than usual, and later on, too, when your 'bump' gets larger and heavier, and the baby gets increasingly active whenever you sit down and rest.

Regular bathing will help keep your skin feeling soft and fresh and smelling sweetly. You can relax in a warm bath or have a bracing shower. Many women like to take a shower in the morning to wake them up, and a bath in the evening to help them sleep. It is entirely a matter of personal preference. You may find that showering is easier later on in pregnancy when getting in and out of the bath can pose problems.

Try to develop a bathing routine that suits you – bathe, dry and moisturize, paying special attention to breasts, any areas of dry skin and potential stretch mark zones. Do this daily to keep your skin beautiful. Use your time in the bath relaxing and letting the day's worries slip away.

The right temperature
This is very important indeed when you are pregnant as we shall see. Most of us tend to take too hot a bath which is cumulatively damaging to our skin. Obviously, your decision will be influenced by a combination of factors – the time of day, how you feel, the weather and the benefits you wish to receive. Here is a guide to choosing the right temperature.

1   Hot baths (above 95 °F/34 °C) There are no benefits to be gained from taking a really hot bath. In fact, it will make your skin even dryer than it is already as it causes more of its natural moisture to evaporate. A hot bath can also lead to broken capillaries in the skin and cause you to feel faint or dizzy – never good things during pregnancy. It can also loosen your muscles.

2   Warm baths (85–95 °F/29–34 °C) This is the best temperature range to encourage sleep and relaxation at the end of a tiring day. It helps ease out tired muscles, relieves pain and avoids post-exercise stiffness. Lie back, enjoy the warmth and feel the tension flowing out of your body. It is ideal for aching backs – common in later pregnancy.

3   Tepid baths (75–85 °F/24–29 °C) Perfect in hot weather for cooling you down after a day in the sun, but not really a good idea in winter, this temperature range is reviving and refreshing. It helps induce sleep, too, if the bath is taken immediately before going to bed.

Bath aids
A loofah, massage mit and natural sponge should be prerequisites in every bathroom. Even though you are pregnant you can gently massage your thighs and upper arms to boost circulation and encourage the elimination of skin wastes and toxins. This will help prevent the formation of ugly cellulite which often appears during periods of hormonal changes in the body such as pregnancy.

Fragrant baths
Baths are even more enjoyable when they smell fragrant and sweet. However, you should avoid using bathsalts, foams and harsh soaps if your skin is naturally rather dry. They tend to strip away your skin's natural, protective acid mantle and cause dehydration. Also, if you find that some soaps are irritating to your skin, you should use a mild, non-alkaline pH-balanced soap instead which will not harm you.

In pregnancy the skin has a natural tendency to

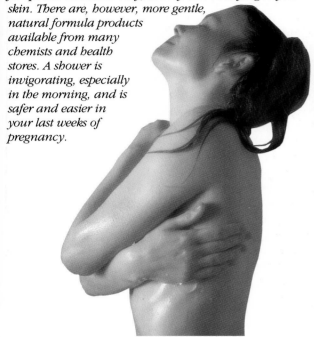

Personal hygiene and feeling clean and fresh are very important during pregnancy. A relaxing bath is soothing at the end of a tiring day, especially if your muscles are aching. Foam baths are luxurious but should be saved for special occasions only, as they can be drying to your skin. There are, however, more gentle, natural formula products available from many chemists and health stores. A shower is invigorating, especially in the morning, and is safer and easier in your last weeks of pregnancy.

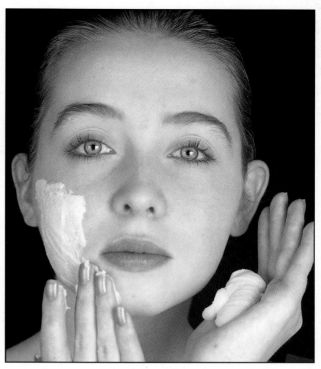

After a bath, when your skin is tingling and clean, rub some moisturizing cream into your face and body to keep them smooth and supple. Apply lightly with your fingertips, especially to delicate areas such as around the eyes.

become dry and rather itchy. When you bathe, add a few drops of fragrant oil to the bath water to moisturize your skin. Oils come in a wide range of fragrances of flowers, herbs and fruits. Find one that you like best. Another remedy for dry skin is to rub a little vegetable oil all over your body before you bathe. This oily coating will help prevent the skin drying.

Softening baths

To keep skin smooth and silky soft you can try adding various oils to the water – lime blossom, lavender, walnut, jasmine, patchouli and rose are all lovely. The ancient Egyptians used to bathe in asses milk. This is probably impractical for you! However, you can try a modern variation for softening dry skin by adding a cup of dried non-fat instant milk to the bath water. Mixing in a few drops of aromatic oil will give it a sweet-smelling fragrance.

Soothing baths

A herbal bath is therapeutic and soothing. Just tie an infusion of fresh herbs in a piece of cheesecloth or muslin and immerse the bag in the bath water under the running tap. Soothing herbs to choose from

include comfrey, lavender, rosemary, sage, marjoram and thyme. Don't throw the bag away afterwards – hang it until the herbs lose their natural fragrance. Fruit, spices and flowers can also be used – try orange or lemon peel, rose petals or cloves.

Bathtime safety

Buy a non-slip rubber bath mat with suction pads on the underside and place in your bath or shower cubicle to prevent slipping. As your 'bump' grows larger and your centre of gravity shifts further forwards, the weight of the baby may throw you off balance as you climb in and out of the bath. It is also very easy to slip on a piece of wet soap, so do take precautions both for your sake and that of the baby.

It may be better in the last few weeks to take a shower instead of a bath. Not only are you less likely to slip but you can avoid the difficulties of getting in and out of the bath, and you will also notice if your waters break. You should be careful not to get so relaxed in the bath that you drift off to sleep. You may wake up cold later on, or find yourself slipping down under the water.

Stay fresh and be a bathing beauty

After bathing

After patting yourself gently dry with a towel – don't rub vigorously if you have dry skin – you can treat yourself to a gentle massage while your skin is still warm and receptive. This not only helps relieve dry, itchy skin but also helps prevent stretch marks. Use a readily absorbed oil or moisturizing cream and smooth it gently into the skin, paying special attention to the abdomen, hips, thighs and breasts. Moisturizing is a very important part of your daily bathing routine as you have fewer oil glands in your body skin than on your face. Don't neglect it. If you suffer from poor circulation you can try rubbing yourself with a soft towel to increase blood flow.

Bathing itself will not replace moisture in your skin – on the contrary, it has the opposite effect and actually dehydrates it. Keep a jar or bottle of fragrant moisturizing lotion beside the bath and smooth it in automatically afterwards.

Perspiration

We all want to smell sweet but you may find that you perspire more than usual during pregnancy. This is caused by the hormone progesterone in your body making your temperature rise. Your body's normal reaction in order to cool itself down is to perspire. The perspiration itself is odourless but the action of bacteria can create unpleasant odours. Bathing every day will help keep skin fresh and clean and remove any bacteria that cause odour. In order to avoid body odour and reduce perspiration you should adhere to the following basic rules:
1   Have a daily bath.
2   Shave your underarms regularly.
3   Use a combined deodorant-antiperspirant.
4   Wear natural fibres such as cotton, linen, silk and wool that allow the skin to breathe.
5   Wear loose, comfortable clothes so that the air can circulate freely around your body.
6   After bathing, apply a dusting of talcum powder to the inner thighs and underarms.
Before you get dressed in the morning or go to bed at night, you should apply a deodorant or antiperspirant. You can choose from roll-ons,

lotions, creams and aerosol sprays, either unperfumed or in a wide range of fragrances. Wait until you are cool and any dampness has disappeared before applying. They are most effective used on hairless skin so shave regularly under your arms or use a depilatory cream. Wait for the product to dry thoroughly before dressing to avoid stains on clothing.

Deodorants work by restricting the action of bacteria on the skin but they may cause reactions if you have sensitive skin.

Antiperspirants reduce perspiration flow as well as fighting the bacteria. However, these too may sometimes cause allergic reactions. If you perspire a lot, you can buy a special long-lasting formula extra-dry antiperspirant which will help keep you dry and odour-free throughout the day, even in the hottest weather. However, if you are allergic to chemicals, you can use green leaves instead. Spinach, herbs, mint and beet tops can all be rubbed under the arms after bathing and drying and will help eliminate perspiration and odour the natural way.

Stretch marks

These sometimes appear in the form of unsightly red lines on the breasts, abdomen, hips and thighs of some pregnant women. Although they eventually fade to silvery-white streaks after delivery, they never disappear completely and thus the best cure is prevention. Why do they occur? Well, they are caused by the elastic fibres in the tissues underlying the epidermis stretching beyond their capacity to the point of rupture.

There seem to be two different kinds of stretch marks during pregnancy:
1   Those caused by hormonal changes in early pregnancy.
2   Those that appear in the last trimester as the skin of the breasts, hips, thighs and abdomen are stretched and distended by the enlarged uterus. Although doctors do not know why, some women seem to have a greater propensity to stretch marks than others. It also appears that older women suffer less than younger mums – perhaps this is because their skin has more 'give'!

Avoiding stretch marks

You can take positive steps to avoid stretch marks or at least to minimize the risk by doing the following:
1   Wear a well-fitting bra which will help prevent your breasts sagging.

2 Gain weight within the safe limits laid down (between 28 and 32lb). Excessive weight gain or too little weight gain can both predispose you to stretch marks.

3 Improve your diet: healthy nutrition is essential for maintaining elastic tissues. You need protein, vitamin C, zinc and vitamin B6 to protect the skin's collagen fibres and keep them strong and supple. Zinc is particularly important in prevention – although it is present in many foods naturally, processing, soil exhaustion and poor cooking methods combine to rob many of the foods we eat of this vital mineral. Taking a zinc supplement, eating organically grown vegetables and cereals and fresh seafood will give you adequate zinc in the diet.

Women who have been taking oral contraceptives are often deficient in zinc and B6 and they should take special care to ensure that they get the recommended daily amounts – 20mg of zinc and 2.6mg of vitamin B6.

4 Many women point to vitamin E as the wonder vitamin for stretch marks prevention but there is little scientific evidence at present to support this. However, there is no harm in taking a supplement as you need it anyway and it may just do the trick for you. You can also smooth oils and lotions containing vitamin E into the skin.

5 You can apply many creams, lotions and ointments externally to keep your skin smooth and supple. Although there are many specially formulated products for prevention on the market, almost any aromatherapy oil, vitamin E cream or lanolin will be effective at keeping skin smooth. Massage these gently into the skin after bathing. But be aware that although they will certainly soften the skin externally they cannot alter the elasticity of the tissues underneath.

6 Another way of boosting the zinc in your body may be to use a zinc-based cream and rub it gently into your skin.

7 Regular exercise will help strengthen the underlying muscles which support the body, and may be beneficial in prevention.

8 Some doctors think that exposing the skin to the sun may also help prevent stretch marks – try it if you are expecting a summer or autumn baby, but be sure to use a protective sunscreen to prevent burning.

If you take all these measures, you will certainly reduce your chances of getting stretch marks. Diet is the most important preventative step you can take and if you are eating a healthy, wholefoods diet you are probably getting all the nutrients you need. However, do be aware that the pregnancy hormones in your body may weaken the elastic fibres in your skin despite all this. You can only do your best and hope that good skincare and healthy diet will keep these ugly scars away.

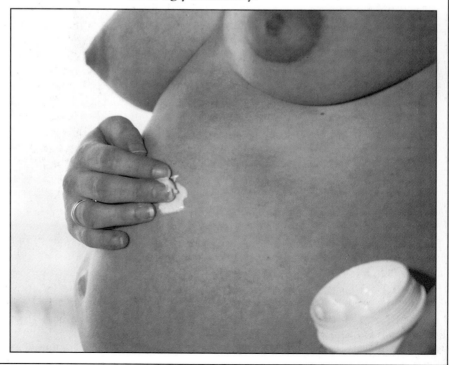

Daily moisturizing of your abdomen will help prevent you developing stretch marks and also relieve any dryness or itchiness caused by the tightness of your skin. After bathing, gently massage some specially formulated moisturizing cream or oil into your stomach area.

Start the day with a nutritious breakfast

Eat a good breakfast

While you are pregnant, breakfast is probably the most important meal of the day, especially in the early months when you may fall prey to morning sickness. Blood sugar levels drop after many hours of not eating – for example, between an early evening meal and breakfast the following day. If you try to skip breakfast you could be creating problems for yourself, and you may feel weak, tired and maybe even faint or dizzy later in the morning.

Even if you are not accustomed to eating breakfast, it is never too late to start. If you are worried about extra calories and putting on too much weight, pause for a minute and consider this. The calories from the food you eat at breakfast are burned up more efficiently by your body as you busy yourself throughout the day than those from the evening meal after which you just relax. Breakfast provides you with energy and stamina for the day – essential when you might be feeling a little below par. Research has shown that we can concentrate better and perform most tasks and jobs more effectively after eating breakfast. People who go without are more likely to have diminished concentration and to feel weary.

The old adage goes, 'breakfast like a king, lunch like a prince, and eat supper like a pauper' but to do this you don't have to indulge in a big traditional fry-up. In fact, if you are inclined to be nauseous, then a fried breakfast of bacon and eggs is probably the worst thing you can eat. Anything fatty or acidic (and that includes your favourite glass of orange juice) may upset your stomach, so it is best to choose more bland alternatives if this is the case.

It is essential that breakfast should supply you with some wide-ranging nutrients, especially protein. This is because it is broken down by your body into amino acids which help stimulate hormones that promote feelings of well-being, and regulate blood sugar levels. Here's how you can get some important nutrients at breakfast-time:

1   Protein

Whole-grain cereals such as muesli, granola, Shredded Wheat and Weetabix will provide some protein. Whole-grain bread or muffins are also a good source, as are eggs (preferably poached, boiled or scrambled if your tummy is delicate), baked beans, bacon, sausages, kidneys, kippers, smoked haddock or ham. The milk or yoghurt that you pour over your breakfast cereal will also supply protein, as will a special high-protein pep-up drink.

2   B vitamins

You will get these from eating vitamin enriched breakfast cereals, whole-grain bread, milk, eggs, banana (good sliced up on top of muesli or whizzed in the blender with milk and yoghurt), bacon and brewers yeast.

3   Vitamin C

Start the day with half a grapefruit (minus the sugar), a glass of fruit juice or some freshly squeezed lemon juice mixed with sparkling mineral water. Other ways of getting vitamin C include soaking your muesli in fruit juice or topping it with chopped fresh oranges, strawberries and grapefruit.

4   Iron

You don't have to eat liver for breakfast to get some iron, you will be relieved to hear. Eggs are a good source, too, and many commercial breakfast cereals are enriched with iron.

5   Fibre

Although fibre is not a nutrient, it is highly desirable in the diet of any pregnant woman to help remove toxins and prevent constipation, piles and varicose veins. Whole-grain bread, cereals, fruit and baked beans will all provide a reasonable breakfast amount.

Home-made versus commercial cereals

Both have their merits as long as the commercial cereals are not heavily sugared and salted. With home-made cereals, you have the benefit of knowing exactly what the ingredients are and being able to vary them according to your mood and taste. However, the muesli and granola you make in your kitchen do not contain all the minerals and B vitamins of many reinforced commercial brands. But they are cheaper, especially if you make them up in bulk and store them in airtight jars or containers. You can add nutrients by serving them with chopped fresh fruit, yoghurt, ground nuts, seeds, milk powder and soaked dried fruits.

When you buy commercial cereals check the

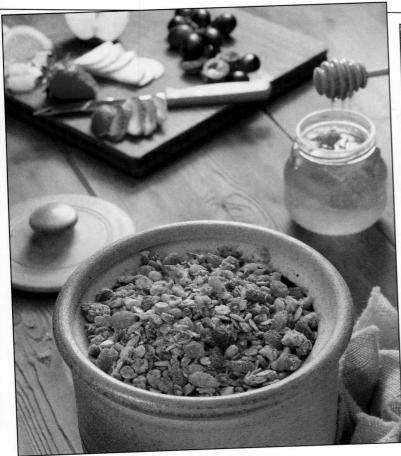

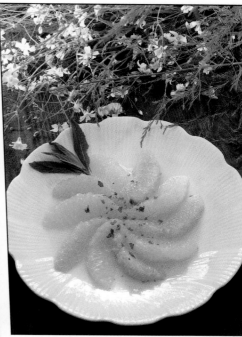

Breakfast is probably the most important meal of all. A fruit salad is nutritious, tasty and easy to make and granola (left) or muesli are good high-fibre ways to begin the day. Try them with milk or yoghurt and for variety add nuts and fresh or dried fruit.

labels carefully. Avoid any that are high in sugar – they only provide unwanted calories and often tend to be lower in other nutrients, too. Many of the 'health' cereals – muesli, bran flakes, hot oat and bran cereals – are supplemented with vitamins and minerals.

Muesli

350g/12oz/4 cups jumbo oats
75g/3oz/3/4 cup rye flakes
50g/2oz/2/3 cup bran
25g/1oz/1/3 cup wheatgerm
100g/4oz/2/3 cup raisins
100g/4oz/2/3 cup chopped dried dates
50g/2oz/1/2 cup chopped hazelnuts
50g/2oz/1/2 cup chopped walnuts
25g/1oz/1/4 cup chopped cashew nuts
50g/2oz/1/2 cup chopped Brazil nuts
50g/2oz/3/8 cup chopped dried apricots

Mix all the ingredients together and store in a large airtight container. Serve as a breakfast cereal or as a

dessert with milk, yoghurt and fresh fruit. Makes approximately 1kg/2lb muesli.

Granola

300g/11oz/3²/3 cups jumbo oats
50g/2oz/²/3 cup bran
25g/1oz/1/3 cup wheatgerm
50g/2oz/1/2 cup chopped hazelnuts
100g/4oz/11/4 cups dessicated coconut
2.5ml/1/2 teaspoon salt
50g/2oz sesame seeds
100ml/4floz/1/2 cup vegetable oil
100ml/4floz/1/2 cup honey
2-3 drops vanilla essence
150g/5oz/3/4 cup raisins
50g/2oz/1/2 cup chopped Brazil nuts
30ml/2 tablespoons chopped cashew nuts

Mix the jumbo oats, bran, wheatgerm, hazelnuts, coconut, salt and sesame seeds in a large bowl. Heat the oil and honey together in a small pan over a low

Start the day with a nutritious breakfast

heat until thoroughly blended. Add the vanilla essence and pour over the granola mixture. Mix well so that all the nuts, grains and seeds are well-coated.

Spread this mixture over a shallow baking tin and bake in a preheated oven at 140°C, 275°F, gas 1 for 35-40 minutes, stirring occasionally. Cool the granola, stir in the raisins, Brazil and cashew nuts and store in an airtight container. Makes approximately 1kg/2lb granola.

Cooked breakfasts

French toast

2 medium eggs, beaten
15ml/1 tablespoon milk or water
salt and pepper
pinch cinnamon (optional)
2 slices 100 per cent wholemeal bread
30ml/2 tablespoons oil

Beat the eggs with the milk or water and seasoning. Add the cinnamon if wished. Place the bread in this mixture and leave to soak up the liquid, turning so that both sides are evenly coated. Heat the oil in a pan and fry the bread until golden. Turn and fry the other side until crisp. For a sweet variation, you can add a good pinch of sugar to the soaking mixture and omit the seasoning. Serve with maple syrup or a little cinnamon sugar and fresh fruit in the American manner. Makes 2 servings.

Scrambled eggs

2 medium eggs
30ml/2 tablespoons milk
salt and pepper
small knob butter or margarine

Beat together the eggs, milk and seasoning with a whisk or fork. Melt the butter over low heat and pour in the scrambled egg mixture (after adding the flavouring of your choice, if used – see below). Stir over low heat until the eggs start to set and 'scramble' – they should be thick, moist and creamy. Do not allow to become too dry nor too watery. Makes 1 serving.
Note: scrambled eggs are delicious served in large fried mushrooms.

Suggested flavourings:
1 few snipped fresh chives or other herbs
2 2 chopped crisply grilled bacon rashers
3 1 small tomato, skinned and chopped
4 50g/2oz finely chopped ham
5 few mushrooms, fried and chopped
6 a little chopped smoked salmon and dill
7 50g/2oz flaked Finnan haddock and chopped parsley
8 5ml/1 teaspoon bran and chopped fresh herbs

Omelette

2 medium eggs
10ml/2 teaspoons cold water
salt and pepper
15g/½oz butter or margarine

Beat the eggs, water and seasoning with a fork – just lightly. Melt the butter in a non-stick omelette pan and when it is sizzling pour in the omelette mixture. Use a fork or spoon to draw the runny liquid in from the sides to the centre. When nearly set, add the filling of your choice and cook over low heat until set. Fold over or roll up and serve immediately. Makes 1 serving.

Fillings:
1 50g/2oz grated cheese
2 50g/2oz chopped ham
3 30ml/2 tablespoons chopped fresh herbs
4 50g/2oz peeled, cooked prawns
5 50g/2oz sautéed mushrooms, chopped
6 1 courgette and 1 tomato, sautéed
7 60ml/4 tablespoons flaked smoked haddock
8 1 grilled bacon rasher and ½ sliced avocado

Kedgeree

50g/2oz/¼ cup long-grain rice (preferably brown)
100g/4oz flaked, cooked smoked haddock
2.5ml/½ teaspoon curry powder
salt and pepper
1 hard-boiled egg, chopped or sieved

15ml/1 tablespoon chopped parsley
lemon wedges and mango chutney

Cook the rice in boiling salted water until tender but still firm. Drain and while still hot mix in the haddock, flavourings, egg and parsley. Serve hot with mango chutney garnished with lemon wedges. Makes 1 serving.

If you don't like preparing breakfast . . .

Well, you can always have a bowl of whole-grain cereal or a high-protein drink. This can be prepared the night before and stored in the refrigerator in an airtight container overnight, ready to pour out the next day. Even a piece of toasted wholemeal bread or a split muffin spread with honey or peanut butter and served with a glass of milk is highly nutritious and better than nothing. Or empty a carton of low-fat 'live' yoghurt into a bowl and mix in some chopped fresh or dried fruit, a handful of nuts and seeds, a little muesli or granola, and you have a satisfying meal. Top with honey.

But perhaps the easiest breakfast of all which can be downed quickly if you are in a hurry is a meal in a glass like a pep-up protein drink. This can also be drunk throughout the day, between meals or whenever you feel weak and hungry.

Drinks and fruit salads

Citrus fruit salad

1 large grapefruit
1 large ruby red grapefruit
3 oranges
juice of ½ lemon
juice of 2 oranges

Remove all the peel and white pith from the grapefruit and oranges with a sharp knife. Carefully divide the fruit into segments, discarding any membranes, pith and pips. Place in a bowl or airtight container and squeeze over any excess juice together with the lemon and orange juice. Serve chilled. Yoghurt is a good accompaniment. This is a very refreshing way to start a new day as long as you do not suffer from morning sickness, in which case it may be too acidic. Makes 2-3 servings.

High protein drink

225ml/8floz/1 cup milk
30ml/2 tablespoons non-instant low-fat milk powder
few drops vanilla essence
5ml/1 teaspoon brewers yeast powder
1 banana or large slice pineapple or berry fruits, mashed or chopped
15ml/1 tablespoon honey (optional)
15ml/1 tablespoon protein powder (optional)
1 egg, beaten

Put all the ingredients in a liquidizer and blend until smooth. You can alter the ingredients as you wish to find the combination you like best. For example, you might try adding wheatgerm, bran, molasses, apple juice, orange segments, peaches, apricots or nectarines. Makes 1 large serving or 2 small ones.

Dried fruit compôte

450g/1lb/3 cups mixed dried fruit (prunes, apricots, peaches, pears, figs, apple rings)
grated rind and juice of ½ lemon
2.5cm/1in cinnamon stick
a little clear honey (optional)

Put all the dried fruit in a large bowl. Cover with water and leave to soak overnight. Transfer to a saucepan with the soaking liquid, the lemon rind and juice, cinnamon and honey if used. Bring to the boil, then reduce the heat, cover with a lid and simmer very gently for about 45-60 minutes until tender. The addition of honey will make the liquid very syrupy. Serve warm or cold for breakfast (or as a dessert) with thick yoghurt. Makes 4 servings.

Early riser yoghurt drink

300ml/½pint/1¼ cups milk
150ml/¼ pint/⅝ cup natural yoghurt
100g/4oz fresh fruit (strawberries, peaches, nectarines, blackberries, raspberries, pineapple, apricots etc) or 1 small banana
honey to taste (optional)

Blend all the ingredients in a blender until very well mixed and smooth. Store in the refrigerator until needed. Makes 3 servings.

Embark on your pregnancy work-out

Basic exercises

By now you should be performing some basic pregnancy exercises every day. Here are a few simple ones to start you off which you can practise right through your pregnancy. They concentrate on the pelvic floor muscles and stomach muscles and will help strengthen these areas. The former are particularly important during labour and for getting back to normal after your baby is born.

Pelvic floor muscles

You may not even realise that you have these muscles but you will hear a lot about them during pregnancy. They support your uterus, bladder and rectum and work very hard during labour when you

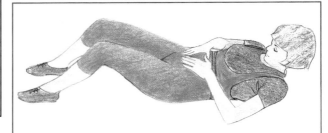

Testing for rectal separation

Lie on your back on the floor with your knees bent and feet flat on the floor, and hip distance apart. Place your hands on your abdomen with the fingers below the navel. Inhale and lift your head and shoulders slightly off the floor, bringing your chin to rest on your chest as you breathe out. You will feel the flesh bulging between the muscles if your rectal muscle has separated.

are pushing the baby through the birth canal. Regular exercise will strengthen them and make them more flexible and elastic. You can test their efficiency when you pass urine. Try interrupting the stream, and then continuing. If you can do this, your muscles are in pretty good shape.

Understanding how these muscles work and exercising to make them strong will enable you to prepare the area for childbirth and reduce the risk of tearing or needing an episiotomy. At antenatal classes you will be taught specially devised exercises to strengthen the pelvic floor. Pelvic tilting is illustrated here. When you do this exercise pay particular attention to your breathing. It will also help you to tone up slack muscles for labour. It also rocks your baby in the pelvic cradle, and thus it is no wonder that newborn babies enjoy being rocked by their mothers in their arms or a cradle and are actually soothed into sleep by the gentle rhythmic motion. Other exercises are:

Pelvic tilting

***1** Lie on the floor with knees bent and slightly apart. Raise buttocks and hips fractionally off the floor and gently roll your pelvis towards chest, exhaling at the same time.*

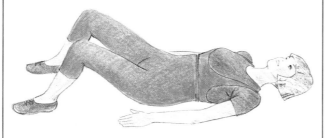

***2** Roll your pelvis back, inhaling as you do so. Relax and lower buttocks to floor. Lift again and roll pelvis slowly around about 20 times.*

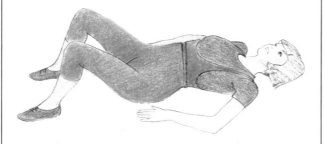

1 Pelvic floor tensing: lie on the floor on your back with your knees bent, feet flat on the floor, and arms at your sides. Slowly tighten the muscles along the rectum and vagina, squeezing upwards and inwards. Inhale slowly and deeply as you contract them and imagine that you are a lift, going up three floors, gradually lifting the muscles upwards through these different stages. Release them gently, exhaling at the same time and repeat 10 times. Although it is restful to practise this exercise lying down, it can also be done standing up, sitting down, lying on your side or even on all-fours. Thus you can practice it anywhere – at work, in the bus queue or lying in bed. Nobody will even notice that you are tensing your pelvic floor muscles!

2 Bridging: lie on your back on the floor with some cushions to support your head and shoulders, and your feet raised and resting on a box or stool. Pull in and tighten your buttocks and the pelvic floor muscles and, keeping your back straight, lift your lower back off the floor. Hold for a count of 10 and then lower your buttocks slowly. Repeat 10 times. This is good for the pelvic floor, abdominal and buttock muscles. It also improves the circulation and blood flow in your legs and helps prevent the formation of unsightly varicose veins.

Abdominal muscles

As your abdomen grows larger it is particularly important to keep the supporting muscles strong to prevent strain on the back and consequent back ache. Bad posture and weak abdominal and back muscles exacerbate the problem. If you thrust your weight too far forwards you will cause these abdominal muscles to sag and distort your spine. Strong abdominal and buttock muscles are the best supportive girdle that you can have during pregnancy. They will help support your baby and your spine. And the stronger and more elastic they are, the more quickly you will regain your figure and a nice flat stomach after the birth of your baby.

Of course, strong abdominal muscles will assist you in labour, too, when you are pushing the baby out along the birth canal. So it is well worth taking care of them and practising the exercises shown and described here regularly – every day if possible. When performing any abdominal exercises, do take care and do not over-strain them or put too much pressure on them. Supporting your head and

Abdominal toner
Lie on floor with feet hip distance apart and knees bent. Cross your arms, exhale and raise head and shoulders and roll up slowly. Hold for a count of 5, pulling in your abdominal muscles and pressing down with hands on either side. Inhale and lower head and shoulders. Repeat 5 times.

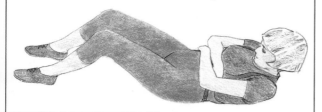

Tummy strengthener
1 Lie on the floor with your knees bent and slightly apart, feet flat on the floor. Support your head and shoulders with a cushion if wished.

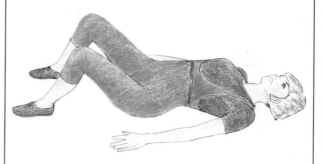

2 Lift your head and shoulders slightly off the floor and reach out with your left hand and touch your right knee. Repeat 10 times.

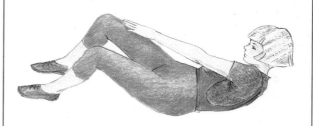

3 Lower yourself to the floor and then repeat on the other side, reaching out with your right hand to touch your left knee. Repeat 10 times.

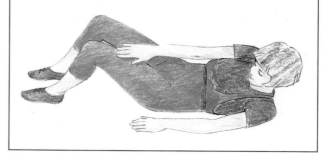

shoulders with thick pillows or cushions will help you to feel more comfortable during the later months of your pregnancy.

Whatever you are doing – whether you are at home, at work, shopping or walking – try to be aware of your abdominal muscles and consciously pull in your abdomen as you exhale. Bracing them regularly in this way helps to strengthen them and

Embark on your pregnancy work-out

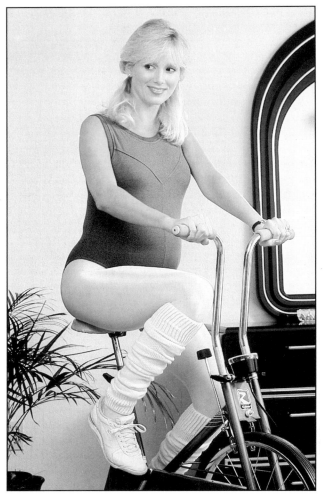

enables you to cope with the increased weight of your enlarged abdomen without putting additional strain on your spine.

Testing for separating of rectus muscle

You must be careful when performing abdominal exercises that you do not separate the rectus muscle. Test for separation by lying on your back, knees bent, feet flat on the floor, and your head supported by a cushion. Rest your hands across your stomach and slowly lift your head and shoulders off the floor, tucking your chin in as you roll up and extending your arms straight out in front of you. Feel your stomach as you do so – the muscle has separated if you can feel a small soft bulge. You may even see the muscle in the later stages of your pregnancy if a thin dark line appears running down through the middle of your navel, although this is not always the case. Avoid leg raises during pregnancy and immediately afterwards as they may also cause separation. Sit-ups are very dangerous and should be left until you have fully recovered and completed a course of post-natal

Exercise rules

Always bear the following points in mind whenever you exercise.

1 Make exercise part of your regular daily routine. Try to set aside the same time every day when you walk, run, work-out, swim or just perform a few simple antenatal exercises.

2 You may find it beneficial to vary the exercise as it can become very boring if it is too repetitive. Try swimming twice a week, an antenatal class on a couple of evenings, a cycle ride at weekends or a long walk in the local park or countryside.

3 Always check that you are performing exercises correctly. If one hurts or causes you any discomfort, stop immediately and concentrate on other ones instead. Never be tempted to 'go for the burn' during pregnancy or to push yourself beyond your physical limits. Be aware that pregnancy may impose certain limitations on what you can achieve and you will have to lower your sights a little. Over-exercising can be dangerous to you and your baby.

4 Build up slowly and gradually, increasing the repetitions and the length of an exercise session only if you get stronger.

exercises. If the muscle does separate it is not necessarily for ever. You can prevent any further separation and you can rehabilitate and strengthen the muscle after birth.

1 Leg sliding: this is good exercise to tone up weak abdominal muscles in a gentle way. Lie on your back, head and shoulders supported by a cushion, knees bent and feet flat on the floor. Make sure that the small of your back is pressed into the floor. Gently lower and slide your legs down to the floor and, keeping your back flat on the floor, slowly raise one knee and then the other. Repeat 10 times.

2 Kneeling strengthener: kneel on the floor with knees slightly apart and arms stretched up above your head. Now smoothly lower both your arms down to the right, twisting at the waist, and touch your feet behind. Raise your arms slowly and repeat to the left. Repeat 10 times each side.

Take care of your stomach

Pregnancy is not the time for practising sit-ups and other strenuous exercises that may put excessive strain on your abdominal muscles. Only practise the recommended exercises and do not be tempted to

Even with your 'bump' you can still exercise regularly. Try varying the exercises you do to prevent boredom; work-outs are excellent as they strengthen specific muscle groups.

perform more repetitions than are necessary. Be prepared for the fact that your abdomen is going to expand. You are exercising these muscles to strengthen and tone them to support your growing baby and enlarged uterus – not to lose weight in this area. Of course, if your muscles are well-conditioned and in good shape, and you exercise regularly then you are less likely to store unwanted fat around your abdomen, hips and waist.

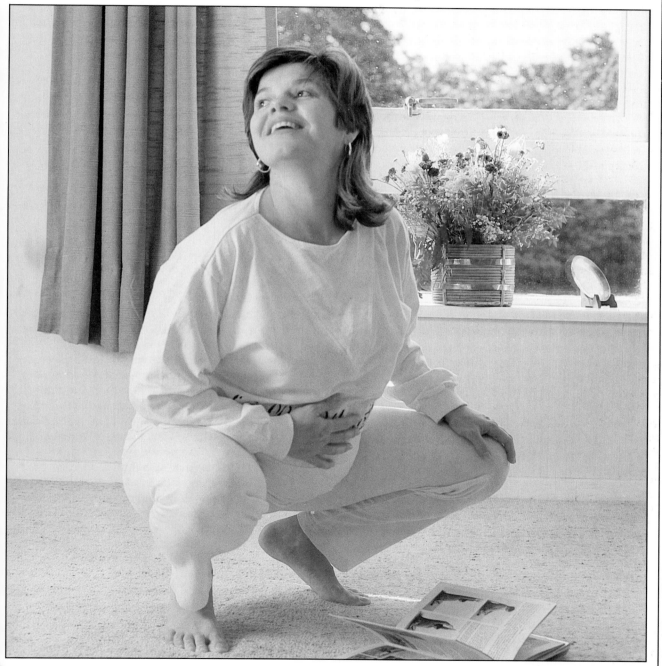

How to choose the sort of birth you want

Your right to choose

You may find that pregnancy and childbirth are a time of self-discovery – when you really get to know the workings of your own body. It should be an enjoyable, fulfilling experience but some women complain that the attitude of doctors, midwives and consultants is obstructive, unsympathetic or even hostile. It is your right to choose the kind of medical care and birth you want, and you should look at the options available in your area and talk to the medical professionals, your family and friends who have had children before taking a decision.

Visiting the clinic

The vast majority of women (98 per cent in the United Kingdom) deliver their babies in hospital. As soon as your pregnancy is confirmed, the machinery will be set in motion to make a booking appointment for you at a hospital antenatal clinic. In your first visit, the arrangements will be made to book you in for the delivery of your baby. The EDD (estimated delivery date) will be calculated, and you will be asked to give details of your medical history – be frank and open about this and do not attempt to conceal anything. Medical staff are quite unshockable and any information you give them may be relevant to the birth and their management of it.

Use this opportunity to ask any questions you may have about pain relief, hospital policy on induction, natural labour etc. If the answers seem unsatisfactory or you are worried about the facilities available or the methods of delivery commonly used, you should try to find out about other hospitals in your area.

You will probably be asked to take a urine sample with you for testing for protein (a symptom of kidney problems or pre-eclampsia), bacteria (possible urinary infection) and glucose (pre-diabetic condition). A blood test will be taken to establish your blood group and whether you have ever had rubella (German measles) which can harm the baby if contracted in the early months of pregnancy. Your blood pressure will be taken and

you will be weighed and measured. You may also be given an internal examination, and your breasts will be examined.

You will be expected to attend the clinic regularly for check-ups on your progress throughout the coming weeks. The arrangements are usually once every four weeks until the twenty-eighth week, then once every fortnight until the thirty-sixth week and weekly thereafter until the birth. Of course, if clinic visits are very difficult for you, perhaps due to transport problems or work commitments, it may be possible to have a similar arrangement with your doctor instead, after the initial booking appointment, although you will still be expected to see the consultant to whom you have been assigned.

In Britain, every pregnant woman is given a 'co-operation' card on which the medical details of her pregnancy are recorded. These include your relevant medical history, results of any tests and screenings and general information about your health. You will be asked to take this card with you to all appointments and, in the last months, to carry it with you at all times in case you go into labour!

You and your doctor

You may be lucky enough to have a good relationship with your doctor, and feel able to discuss any problems or worries with him (her). However, many women complain that their real needs and fears are not understood and that they do not receive all the information they need to know. Male doctors in particular may treat them as helpless, dependent members of the weaker sex, expect them to be unquestioning and passive, and do as they are told meekly. A common complaint among women is that doctors fail to treat them as people and address them face to face – instead, they tend to respond only to their condition and address themselves directly to the women's stomachs.

If this is your problem, you do not have to persevere to develop a better relationship with your doctor – it is possible to change doctors and you can find out how to do this from the Patients Association in the United Kingdom (see the addresses section at the back of this book).

Many women have a better relationship with their midwife than they do with their doctor. She may be more sympathetic and have more time to talk about your pregnancy, the forthcoming delivery and babycare.

If you are over 30 years old, your doctor may describe you rather unflatteringly as an 'elderly primagravida' although you still feel young, fit and attractive. It may be something of a shock to be treated as a freak or an older woman at the ripe old age of, say, 35, especially if you are in the best of health! Nowadays, there is no need to feel unusual or different just because you have opted to have a baby in your thirties. This is becoming increasingly common as more women wait to start a family until they have established themselves in their careers and found some measure of financial and emotional security. Of course, the risks associated with pregnancy, childbirth and the baby's health increase the older one gets, but a healthy lifestyle, modern medical care and methods of testing and screening for abnormalities make later pregnancies a relatively safe and sensible choice. Do not be intimidated by the doctors or nurses who infer that you are too old to be a mother. On the contrary, many new mothers in their thirties claim that they are pleased they waited and that they are more tolerant, patient and understanding than they would have been had they had their babies in their twenties.

What sort of birth

You still have plenty of time to think about the kind of delivery you want and whether you wish to opt for a controlled birth in hospital or a more comfortable, informal one at home. There is no doubt that you will be encouraged and advised to go to hospital, especially if this is your first baby or if you have had difficult labours in the past. And although you are legally entitled to deliver at home and your local authority has a duty to provide a midwife, if any complications were to arise, you would have to be transported immediately to the nearest hospital for specialized treatment. Obviously, this would pose considerable risks to the health of your baby as well as yourself.

So the pros and cons of a home delivery have to be weighed very carefully against those of a hospital delivery, where the atmosphere may be less comfortable and more sterile, but skilled help is always on hand should it be needed. Highly trained medical staff can perform emergency Caesarean sections and offer sophisticated pain relief and monitoring. Also, your baby can be examined immediately after the birth by a qualified paediatrician and you can have a rest before you return home. If you are a first-time mum you can learn how to look after your baby and receive help and encouragement in establishing breastfeeding.

The next question to resolve is whether you wish

to have a natural delivery without any drugs and medical intervention or want to opt for some form of pain relief. Most women wish to be in control of their labours and their bodies, fully conscious throughout and able to participate fully in the birth experience. But however well-intentioned and high-principled you may be about wanting a natural delivery, you may find that the pain, especially in a backache or complicated labour, is difficult to bear, and it is sensible to consider the various forms of pain relief available before you go into labour. Even at this early stage in your pregnancy when you are being booked into a hospital, you should ask whether epidurals are offered if needed (a skilled anaesthetist has to administer them) and what is the hospital's attitude to drugs and pain relief, natural birth, induction, birthing stools etc.

You can feel confident throughout your pregnancy if you understand how your body works and are not afraid to ask questions about delivery and birth.

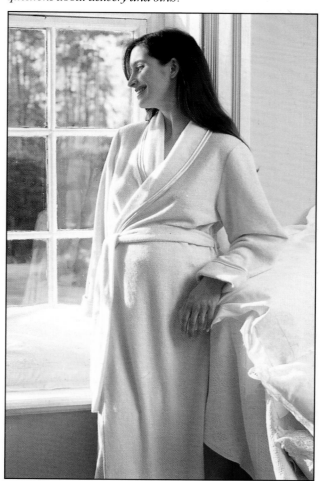

Feel your baby move at last

You

This month you will begin to look pregnant as well as feeling your baby move for the first time. Although you will not have a real 'bump', your tummy will start to look more rounded and your waist will be thickening significantly. You may have problems doing up zip fasteners and buttons on jeans and skirts. However, it is probably still too early to start wearing flowing maternity clothes. Just wear some of your looser tops, dresses and dungarees or jumpsuits. You may wish to start making some looser clothes for the coming months or looking at the ranges of maternity wear available in the boutiques and chainstores. You will be pleasantly surprised at how fashionable and colourful they are.

Although you may still feel tired in the evenings you are probably fired up with new energy and any extreme feelings of fatigue or nausea will have disappeared for good. Now is the time to start watching your weight gain. This does not mean that you should actively try to keep your weight down to its present level or eat low-calorie foods – this might endanger your baby's health. On the contrary, you must eat sensibly and avoid foods that are high in calories and low in goodness, like cakes, biscuits, puddings and sweets. See the table on page 84 for what constitutes a sensible weight gain.

A dark line may now appear down the centre of your abdomen from the navel or even higher to the pubic area. Don't worry – this is the *linea nigra*. It will disappear after the baby is born. You might also notice the first signs of stretch marks (*see* page 51 for advice on how to avoid them or prevent them getting worse). Although they fade to a pale silver after delivery they are best avoided if possible. Another common development in the fourth month, usually after week 16, is the appearance of colostrum. This is a clear fluid which is expressed from the breasts during pregnancy and is the ideal highly nutritious food for your baby in the first few days of life before the milk flow establishes itself. One body of medical opinion holds that it is beneficial to express it regularly in order to clear the milk ducts. However, some doctors advise you not to do this as there might be only a limited supply. Ask *your* doctor for advice.

You should be caring for your breasts every day now – washing them and gently smoothing in some moisturizing cream or a special anti-stretch mark preparation. Creams and lotions that contain lanolin or vitamin E are often very effective. You will also need a firm support bra as they get larger and heavier, if they are to keep their shape and firmness.

The most exciting moment will be when you actually feel your baby move inside you. This may happen any time after the sixteenth week. At first it will feel like little fluttering butterfly sensations in your tummy but they will get stronger very quickly. This is known as 'quickening' and you are now aware of the physical reality of the baby inside you.

Your baby

Although your baby only weighs 150g/5oz, she is developing fast by the end of the fourth month. She has eyebrows and hair on her head and she looks a little more human every day. At the moment she is covered with fine downy hair known as *lanugo*. In her mouth, the two halves of her palate have fused together, and the bone cores are growing out to replace the gristle in her skeleton. Her bones will not stop developing, in fact, until she is twenty-five years old. Her eyes are closed as the eyelids grew together during the third month and do not open again until the seventh month of pregnancy.

An ultrascan picture now might reveal that your baby is already beginning to suck her thumbs. Whenever she draws her thumb close to her mouth her lips and tongue will automatically start their sucking motion. This is one of the earliest reflexes, and perhaps it is comforting even at this early stage. Inside the womb the baby kicks her legs, waves her arms and grasps. She can hear the pounding of your pulse, the murmuring of the placenta and even your voice. Sometimes the placenta surges as you move suddenly. So her existence is not totally silent and still. She exists in a moving, relatively noisy environment. Perhaps this is why some mothers play their babies tapes of 'womb noises' to comfort them and get them to sleep after they are born.

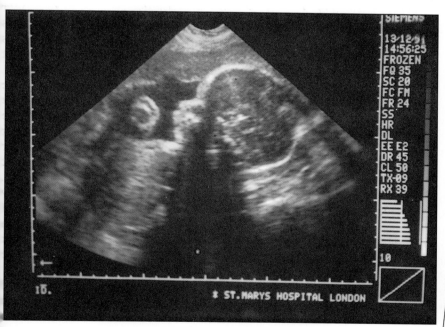

This is a typical ultrasound scan picture. As you can see, you will be disappointed if you expect a clear view of your baby inside the womb. Although it is intelligible to the trained eye, the scan operator will have to point out the features and the limbs.

Take a look at your baby

Often in the fourth month of pregnancy you are given an ultrasound scan to establish the delivery date and check up on your baby's progress. This is a marvellous opportunity to actually see the baby inside you. To the untrained eye, a scan may appear blurred but when the operator explains the picture on the screen to you and helps you to distinguish the sometimes confusing shapes and images, it can be a very exciting experience. If you are lucky, you might even see your baby kicking her legs or sucking her thumb. If you thought that it would enable you to discover the sex of your baby, however, you will be disappointed, but it would show if you were expecting twins, for instance.

Keep your breasts shapely and beautiful

During pregnancy you will become very aware of your breasts and should pay special attention to them. Breasts need regular care and exercise to keep them firm and shapely, to avoid stretch marks and to prepare them for breastfeeding after the birth of your baby. It is all too easy to neglect them in pregnancy and regret it later on.

One of the first signs of pregnancy that you will notice is that your breasts will get fuller and heavier, the nipples may become erect easily and the areolae surrounding the nipples will darken. Small raised lumps called Montgomery's tubercles will probably appear, especially in a first pregnancy, which secrete a lubricant. As your blood flow increases, your breasts may feel tender, sore or tingly and little veins may stand out on them. Apart from missing your period, these are the most obvious indications of your new pregnancy.

Anatomy of breasts

Each breast is a milk-producing mammary gland and is made up of 50 per cent adipose (fatty) tissue and fibrous connective tissue. This fat surrounds the mammary gland itself and determines the shape and firmness of your bosom. The function of the breasts is to produce milk to feed your baby, and from very early on in pregnancy they start preparing for this. How beautiful your breasts are – how they hang, their firmness and shape – is determined partly genetically and also by the care you lavish upon them and whether you wear a well-fitting support bra. Pregnancy and breastfeeding can cause your breasts' natural shape and firmness to change if you do not take adequate care of them.

Choosing a good support bra

A well-fitting support bra will make you feel more comfortable and prevent the ligaments that support the breasts and hold them up stretching and sagging. Once the ligaments and skin do stretch they will

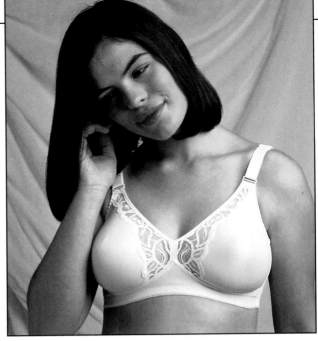

Make sure that your bra is the right size to support your breasts. A front-opening one will be ideal for breastfeeding your baby after birth.

never regain their natural shape so it is well worth taking positive action to avoid this. Prevention is the best cure as always, so invest in a support bra. It need not be cumbersome or ugly – some are very pretty in broderie anglaise or lacy materials – but it should provide adequate support and have wide shoulder straps and an adjustable back so that it will expand as the months go by. Any bras you buy in the last months should be front opening so that you can wear them after the birth for breastfeeding.

When you buy a bra, be sure to try it on and be convinced that it really does feel comfortable. It should not be too tight nor pinch the skin. The straps should fit well over your shoulders without falling down and slipping off, and there should be a band around the lower margin. Many companies make special bras for pregnancy and nursing so look at the ranges and see which models are best for you. As a general rule, cotton is preferable to nylon as it is cooler to wear and you are less likely to perspire.

A good bra will make your breasts feel more comfortable, enable you to exercise with ease and help prevent stretch marks and sagging. Some women find that their breasts get so heavy in later pregnancy that sleeping is difficult without a bra. You can buy a specially designed gentle support bra for sleeping in, too. Whatever bra you buy, make sure that there is room for all-over expansion – they are expensive and you do not want to replace it every month as your bosom gets bigger and bigger.

Caring for your breasts

It is a good idea from early on in pregnancy to develop a daily routine in order to keep breasts clean and supple and to prepare them for breastfeeding. Cleanliness is essential, especially when the breasts start to leak colostrum. You should wash them every day with mild soap and warm water to remove any little crusts. Dry thoroughly, especially the nipple area, and then gently smooth in some soothing cream – a specially formulated one or a lanolin-based product. Some women swear by vitamin E creams for preventing stretch marks and keeping the skin smooth, soft and supple but there is little scientific evidence to support this.

To prepare your breasts for nursing, you must ensure that they are strong and in good shape. Some doctors recommend that if they are very sensitive or your nipples are inverted you should rub them with a wet flannel to toughen them up and to encourage the nipples to stand out of their own accord. If this sounds too rough, don't worry. You can still breastfeed even if you have inverted nipples. Just cream the breasts regularly to keep them soft and free from cracks. You may find that pregnancy often helps the nipples to stand erect anyway, or that when your baby eventually suckles she will do the job for you.

You can encourage the nipples to stand out by pulling them gently forwards in the last couple of months. Hold the nipples between finger and thumb and very gently coax them outwards. Practise this every day. Some doctors and midwives think that wearing breast shells is a good idea in the last month or so. These consist of plastic discs that fit snugly over the breasts and are worn inside your bra. There are holes cut in them to exert pressure on the nipples and encourage them to protrude through the centre of the shell as they become more erect. However, some doctors feel that they put unnecessary pressure on the milk ducts and do not advise their use.

Colostrum

Even before your baby is delivered, you may find that your nipples start to secrete a clear or slightly yellowish fluid called colostrum. This is produced as the first food for your baby. It is highly nutritious as it is a rich source of nutrients and antibodies. It becomes more plentiful after birth and is the ideal nourishment for your baby until the milk flow proper becomes established – usually on the third or fourth day after delivery of the baby.

The colostrum may appear as early as during the second trimester and it is a sure sign that your breasts are getting ready for the job of nursing. However, don't worry if the colostrum does not appear until the last few weeks – the time varies for different women. You can practise expressing it for nursing quite easily. Just place both thumbs above the areola of one breast with the fingertips below. Move them inwards towards the nipple, squeezing gently. Colostrum will be expressed from the breasts. It is unlikely to shoot out and probably only tiny beads will appear. Repeat the exercise with the other breast to empty that, too.

If colostrum does start to leak from your breasts the secretion may dry and go crusty. You must wash it away with soap and water or you are likely to end up with dry, sore, cracked nipples. Either allow your breasts to dry naturally in the air or pat gently dry with a soft towel. Moisturize thoroughly with a soothing cream or lotion.

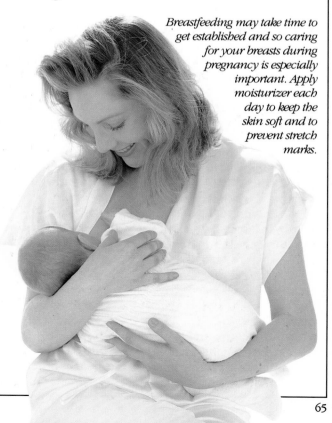

Breastfeeding may take time to get established and so caring for your breasts during pregnancy is especially important. Apply moisturizer each day to keep the skin soft and to prevent stretch marks.

Keep your breasts shapely and beautiful

Exercise your breasts

This may sound strange but it makes good sense if you want to keep your breasts firm and in shape. When you exercise you work the supporting muscles below the breasts and also those in your arms and shoulders – the breasts themselves contain no muscle. Regular exercise not only keeps the breasts shapely and prevents sagging but also makes them function more efficiently.

1 Wall push-ups
Stand with your feet hip distance apart, just over an arm's length away from a wall. Lean forwards and rest your hands, palms down and facing inwards, at shoulder level on the wall. Now slowly lower yourself forwards, bending your arms at the elbows, until your nose just touches the wall. Slowly straighten your arms and push yourself up and away from the wall to leave only your hands resting on it in the starting position. Repeat the exercise at least 10 times. Exhale deeply as you raise your body and inhale as you lower it towards the wall.

2 Seated with books
Sit up straight on a high backed chair with your feet flat on the floor. Hold out your arms to the sides, fully extended, with a moderately heavy book in each hand. Now bend your elbows and slowly bring in the books towards your chest still holding them at shoulder level. Hold for a count of 5 and straighten your arms again. Repeat this exercise 5 times. You can, if you prefer, use telephone directories as Marilyn Monroe was reputed to do. It worked for her, after all, so it's worth a try!

3 Making fists
Sit cross-legged on your sitting bone keeping your back perfectly straight. Now bend your arms and make a fist with one hand and clasp it in the other at breast-level. Press tightly together several times and feel the pull in your pectoral muscles. Change hands and repeat to the other side. Do 5 repetitions with each hand.

4 Small circles
Stand up tall with your feet shoulder distance apart and your arms extended out to the sides at shoulder level. Now fling your arms back and make complete circles backwards 5 times. Then repeat in the other direction forwards 5 times. You can vary the routine by doing it with your palms facing upwards, downwards or outwards.

5 Hand presses
Sit in a cross-legged position with your hands clasped together in front of you at shoulder level and your elbows bent. Now press your hands together as hard as you possibly can. Keep pressing and releasing and feel the muscles at the sides of your body contracting and relaxing. Build up to 10 repetitions.

Diet and your breasts

Just as good diet affects your health, your level of energy, your skin and hair, it also helps keep your breasts firm with elastic tissues. As you know, it is essential for preventing stretch marks and preserving healthy collagen fibres. The nutrients you need for well-shaped, firm breasts with smooth, supple skin are:
1 **Vitamin C** to manufacture collagen. So ensure that you eat adequate amounts of citrus fruit (oranges, tangerines, grapefruits), baked jacket potatoes, peppers, strawberries, blackcurrants and green vegetables.
2 **Vitamin B6** for collagen and smooth skin –

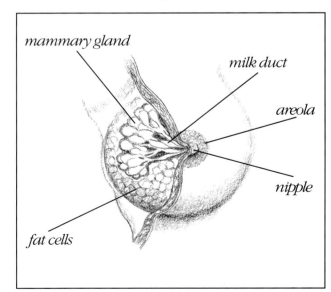

mammary gland

milk duct

areola

nipple

fat cells

available in brewers yeast, whole-grain cereals, offal, meat, eggs and bananas.

3   Zinc to prevent stretch marks. Find it in meat, poultry, dairy products, wholemeal bread and whole-grain cereals.

The quality of your diet will also affect the nutritional content of your breast milk after birth, and if you plan to breastfeed it is essential that you eat a healthy, varied diet both before and after the delivery of your baby. Nutrients are the building blocks for a good milk flow, and if you are malnourished you may experience problems breastfeeding. The more protein, vitamins, minerals and polyunsaturated fats you consume, the more will be present in your milk. So you can see that the quality of your milk will depend on the raw materials you use.

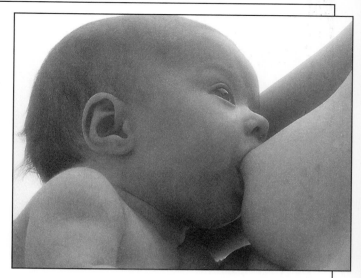

Breastfeeding has many advantages for you and your baby. It helps bond you closer together; it speeds up the process of regaining your figure; it supplies your baby with highly nutritious, anti-infective, non-allergenic milk which is the best start that she can get in life; and it is convenient, effortless and enjoyable for you both.

Why breastfeed?

The old saying goes that 'breast is best' and there is no doubt that breast milk is the best food for your baby in at least the first six months of her life. It is nutritionally superior to commercial formulas and provides the ideal balance of nutrients for your baby with exactly the right proportions of protein, vitamins, minerals, carbohydrate and fat to promote healthy growth and development.

Breast milk is also anti-infective and non-allergenic. Its antibodies help protect your baby against many viral and bacterial infections and build up resistance to disease. Babies who are nursed are less likely to suffer from allergies later on and are often healthier than bottlefed ones. They tend to suffer from fewer infections, have a greater proportion of muscle, less fat and a stronger constitution.

Breastfeeding has advantages for you, too, as it is convenient and labour-saving – saves time spent messing about sterilizing and preparing bottles of feeds. It is always on tap and perfectly free. It also helps you regain your figure more quickly and effectively as the fat stored during pregnancy in preparation for lactation is gradually used up in your

This cross-section through a breast shows the milk ducts through which the milk flows to the nipples for feeding your baby. The breasts consist mainly of fatty tissue and contain no muscles. However, they are supported by muscles and ligaments attached to the ribs, breastbone, upper arm bone and collarbone. When the baby sucks on the nipple, she stimulates milk supply and you experience the 'letdown' of milk.

daily milk production. And, perhaps most important of all, it helps create a strong loving bond between you and your baby. You will cherish some of these quiet moments together and the special closeness that nursing brings.

Don't be disappointed or feel guilty if you cannot breastfeed for some reason or do not wish to do so. The best method is the one you enjoy and feels most comfortable. It is silly to perservere with breastfeeding your baby if you feel unhappy about it – you will both be irritable as a result. Your baby will thrive on formula and you can cuddle her tightly against you as she bottle-feeds to make her feel secure and loved. Above all, don't feel a failure as a mother. You are not. There is more to being a mum than the ability to nurse your baby yourself.

You need not decide now which of the methods you are going to use – there will be plenty of time after the birth to try breastfeeding and discover whether it is right for you and your baby. If you do experience problems and still want to continue nursing your baby, there are several organizations that can help you with representatives and counsellors in your area. These include LaLeche League and the National Childbirth Trust (in the UK). They also have helpful literature on making preparations for breastfeeding which you can send away for.

High-fibre foods for health and beauty

Eat plenty of fibre

We have all heard a lot spoken about fibre recently and it has become a fashionable item in our diet. Fibre is not just a slimming aid as many people seem to think – it also has an important role to play in creating a healthy diet, especially when you are pregnant. So what is fibre?

Fibre is a highly complex cellulose substance which is found in the cells of plants. It is not digestible and thus it cannot be broken down like most foods by enzymes in your body in the usual way. It seems that the human body is actually programmed in some way to deal with the fibre in food, and when it is not present over a long period of time, serious health problems can result.

You need fibre to shunt food quickly through your body; to give it bulk as it passes through the bowel for speedy elimination; and to retain water and eliminate toxins from your system. A high-fibre diet not only helps keep you slim – as you have to chew your food more and feel full-up more quickly – but it also reduces the likelihood of such modern affluent diseases as diverticular disease, colon cancer, hiatus hernia, varicose veins, appendicitis and piles. People who eat highly refined diets, which are low in unprocessed wholefood ingredients, tend to lack essential fibre and to retain food residues in their bodies for longer than the recommended transit time (about two days maximum, preferably one).

Constipation in pregnancy

For many women, constipation is a fact of life, but it really isn't a normal state of affairs. It is a sure signal that you are not functioning as nature intended and that you should change your diet. In pregnancy, straining can lead to the formation of ugly varicose veins in your legs, as it may reduce blood flow. The hormone levels in your body make the situation worse as they cause the vein walls themselves to become slack. Excessive straining can also lead to painful piles, so do make sure that you get enough fibre.

It is best to avoid chemical laxatives which can interfere with your digestion and the absorption of nutrients, irritate the tissues and, in some rare cases, may even be potentially harmful to the baby. Also, do not take mineral oil to relieve constipation as it may cause severe vitamin deficiencies. Regular exercise, such as daily walking, swimming or a pregnancy work-out, will help prevent constipation, and a good diet will work wonders. Here's how to include some high-fibre foods in your diet:

1   Start the day with high-fibre cereal
Muesli, granola, bran flakes, Shredded Wheat, Weetabix and All Bran are all high in fibre. The low-sugar cereals are preferable, and you can always boost their fibre content by sprinkling a tablespoon of natural bran over the top and adding some fibrous sliced fruit – for example, apples, bananas, raspberries, strawberries or figs – or some soaked dried fruit – apricots, prunes, peaches and pears.

2   Eat a fresh salad every day
Not only are salads high in vitamins and minerals but they are rich in fibre, too. You can also eat fresh fruit and salad vegetables as between-meal snacks when you feel like nibbling at something – healthier and less fattening than crisps, chocolate and biscuits.

3   Cut out over-refined starchy foods
Say goodbye to bread, cakes and puddings made with white flour. All the natural fibre, or bran, of the wheat grain is removed in the processing, together with wheatgerm which contains valuable vitamins and protein. Choose bread, pastry, cakes and biscuits that are baked with 100 per cent wholemeal flour. If it is stoneground, better still, for this process ensures that the wheatgerm oil is more evenly distributed throughout the flour.

Most bakers and supermarkets now sell wholemeal bread and rolls, although you should check that they do not contain any unnecessary additives. Or you can bake your own. Health food shops even sell wholemeal biscuits, cakes, cookies, pies and flans.

4   Eat sufficient vegetables
A good source of fibre, especially if eaten with their skins like a baked potato. Beans are also high in fibre – either baked, from a can or soaked and cooked.

5   As a last resort, try prunes
Prunes and other dried fruit are a great natural

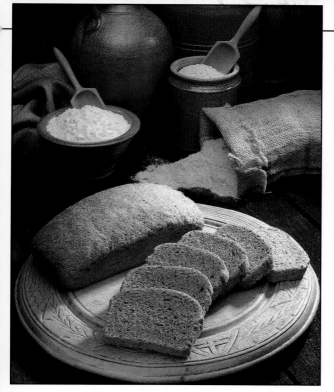

Wholemeal bread is an easy and enjoyable way to increase your fibre intake. Also try pastry, cakes and biscuits baked with 100 per cent wholemeal or stoneground flour.

laxative if you are constipated. Soak them overnight in lemon juice and eat them for breakfast with 'live' natural yoghurt. They will soon start the good work!

Iron tablets can make you constipated

Some women find that iron tablets prescribed by their doctors during pregnancy cause them to become constipated. If this is the case, talk to your doctor about switching to another formula or brand, and do include plenty of fibre-rich foods in your diet. Don't *stop* taking the iron tablets – your baby needs the iron they provide.

Cooking the high-fibre way

It need not be expensive nor difficult to include plenty of high-fibre foods in your diet. Throwing out any bags of white flour and using only wholemeal flour in baking, sauce-making and as a thickening agent is a good starting point. Switching to wholemeal pasta and brown rice from the normal white varieties also helps – these are both sold in supermarkets. Eat plenty of fruit, vegetables and

salads, and try to eat a bean or pulse dish at least twice a week.

High-fibre foods: bran cereals, wholemeal bread, beans and pulses, prunes and dried fruit, peas and sweetcorn, baked potatoes, brown rice, leafy green vegetables, bananas.
Medium-fibre foods: most green vegetables, most breakfast cereals, apples, carrots, nuts, oranges, celery, muesli, wholemeal pasta.
Low-fibre foods: white bread, white rice and pasta, tomatoes, lettuce, cucumber, mashed or boiled potatoes, chips.

Recipes

Here are some high-fibre recipes for you to try out and include in your weekly menus. They all contain high nutritional goodness as well as fibre. Some are suitable for everyday family meals – some can even be served for dinner parties and special occasions. You don't have to suffer or sacrifice flavour to enjoy high-fibre foods!

Soups and starters

Bean and pepper salad

175g/6oz/1 cup kidney beans
1 small red pepper
1 small green pepper
1 onion, thinly sliced in rings
1 spring onion/shallot, chopped
chopped chives
Dressing:
45ml/3 tablespoons olive oil
juice of 1 lemon
15ml/1 tablespoon wine vinegar
salt and pepper

Soak the dried kidney beans overnight and then drain and rinse them. Place in a pan of cold water (do not add salt as this will harden the beans) and bring to the boil. Boil hard for 10 minutes. Drain and rinse the beans and transfer to a pan of fresh cold water. Bring to the boil and simmer for about 1 hour until tender. Drain and cool.

Cut out the core and seeds of the peppers and slice horizontally in thin rings. Place in a salad bowl with the beans and onion.

Mix the dressing and toss with the bean salad and sprinkle with chopped chives. Makes 4 servings.

High-fibre foods for health and beauty

Bean and tomato soup

100g/4oz/⅔ cup red kidney beans, soaked overnight
1 large onion, peeled and chopped
1 large carrot, peeled and chopped
1 clove garlic, crushed
1 small swede or turnip, peeled and diced
30ml/2 tablespoons oil
5ml/1 teaspoon mixed herbs (oregano, basil, chervil or parsley – if you use fresh, double the quantity)
5ml/1 teaspoon turmeric
salt and pepper
4 tomatoes, peeled, seeded and chopped
juice of ½ lemon

Rinse the beans, place in a pan and cover with fresh water. Boil hard for 10 minutes. Strain and rinse the beans. Return to the pan, add sufficient fresh water to cover and bring to the boil. Simmer for 1 hour.

In another pan, fry the vegetables slowly in the oil without colouring for 10 minutes. Add the herbs and turmeric and 550ml/1 pint/2½ cups of water. Bring to the boil, simmer for 15 minutes and then add the cooked beans together with the liquid. Continue cooking until the beans are tender, season to taste and stir in the tomatoes and lemon juice. Cook for a few more minutes to bring out the flavours and then serve with grated cheese if wished. Makes 4 servings.

Main meals

Cowboy baked beans

450g/1lb/2⅔ cups haricot beans
1 large onion, studded with 3 cloves
1 large onion, chopped
15ml/1 tablespoon oil
60ml/4 tablespoons black treacle or molasses

100g/4oz/½ cup soft brown sugar
45ml/3 tablespoons tomato paste
15ml/1 tablespoon Dijon mustard
salt and pepper
225g/8oz salt belly pork or gammon

Soak the beans overnight. Drain and cover with fresh water (approximately 1 litre/1¾ pints/4¼ cups water). Add the clove-studded onion and bring to the boil. Simmer for about 50 minutes or until tender. Drain, reserving the onion and cooking water.

Sauté the onion in the oil until golden. Add the treacle, sugar, tomato paste, mustard, seasoning and 400ml/14floz/1¾ cups of the reserved cooking liquid. Finally, add the whole piece of belly pork or gammon and bring to the boil. Cover the pan and place in a very low preheated oven at 130°C, 250°F, gas ½ for about 3½ hours. Remove the pork and cut into small pieces, discarding any excess fat. Replace in the bean pot and return to the oven, uncovered, for another 30 minutes. Makes 4 servings.

Apricot chicken and rice

225g/8oz/1 cup long-grain brown rice
25ml/5 teaspoons salt
1 onion, finely chopped
30ml/2 tablespoons oil
4 chicken portions, skinned and boned
25g/1oz/2 tablespoons raisins
50g/2oz/⅜ cup dried apricots
30ml/2 tablespoons pine nuts
2.5g/½ teaspoon each ground coriander and cinnamon
salt and pepper
25g/1oz/2 tablespoons margarine
30ml/2 tablespoons chopped fresh parsley

First prepare the rice. Wash in boiling water and then place it in a bowl with 15ml/1 tablespoon salt and cover with cold water. Set aside for a minimum of 2 hours. Drain and rinse the rice and then cook in a pan of boiling water to which the remaining salt has been added, until just tender but still firm. Drain.

Sauté the onion in the oil until it starts to brown. Add the chicken portions and brown on both sides. Next stir in the dried fruit, nuts, spices and seasoning. Pour in enough water to barely cover the chicken, cover the pan and simmer for 1 hour.

Heat the margarine and add half of the cooked

rice. Place the chicken and the sauce on top and cover with the remaining rice. Cover with a clean cloth and a lid and steam over low heat for 25 minutes. Serve immediately sprinkled with parsley.

Chicken and bean risotto

15ml/1 tablespoon oil
1 onion, chopped
2 cloves garlic, crushed
1 red pepper, seeded and sliced thinly
225g/8oz/1 cup long-grain brown rice
150ml/¼ pint/⅝ cup chicken stock
small packet saffron
75g/3oz/½ cup raisins
salt and pepper
225g/8oz chopped, cooked chicken
2 tomatoes, skinned and chopped
100g/4oz button mushrooms, sliced
175g/6oz cooked or canned red kidney beans
30ml/2 tablespoons chopped parsley
grated Parmesan cheese

Heat the oil and sauté the onion and garlic until soft and translucent. Add the red pepper and sauté for 2-3 minutes. Stir in the rice and make sure all the grains are glistening with oil. Add some of the chicken stock and bring to the boil. Sprinkle with saffron to colour the rice golden and add the raisins. Season to taste. Cook over low heat until the rice is plump and tender, adding more stock as and when necessary. When cooked, stir in the chicken, tomatoes, mushrooms and kidney beans and heat through. Serve with parsley and Parmesan. Makes 4 servings.

Puddings

Sweet fruit and pasta pudding

225g/8oz/1½ cups dried fruit (apricots, peaches or pears)
50g/2oz/⅓ cup raisins
225g/8oz wholewheat macaroni
50g/2oz/¼ cup margarine
2 dessert apples, peeled, cored and diced
juice of 1 lemon
50g/2oz/¼ cup soft brown sugar

pinch of ground cloves
2 eggs, separated
25g/1oz/½ cup fresh breadcrumbs
25g/1oz/¼ cup chopped nuts (almonds, walnuts, hazelnuts)

Soak the dried fruit for several hours and drain. Place in a pan, cover with a little water and simmer until tender. Drain and set aside. Soak the raisins in hot water for 30 minutes to plump them up. Cook the macaroni in boiling water for 10 minutes. Drain and mix in the margarine, apple, juice and raisins.

Whisk the sugar, cloves and egg yolk until light and frothy. Whisk the whites until glossy and standing in stiff peaks. Fold into the yolk mixture and gently mix into the cooked macaroni.

Pour the macaroni mixture into a well-greased 900ml/1½pint/3¼ cup ovenproof dish and sprinkle with breadcrumbs and nuts. Dot with a little margarine and bake in a preheated oven at 180°C, 350°F, gas 4 for 30 minutes. Makes 4 servings.

Summer pudding

450g/1lb mixed blackcurrants and other soft fruits
150g/5oz/⅝ cup soft brown sugar
15ml/1 tablespoon crème de cassis
8 slices one-day-old wholemeal bread,
5mm/¼in thick

Put the mixed fruit and sugar in a saucepan and leave overnight (this helps to extract the fruit juices). Next day, bring to the boil and then simmer for 3 minutes. Cool and add the cassis.

Remove the crusts from the bread. Place one slice of bread in the base of a 900ml/1½ pint/3½ cup pudding basin. Cut the other slices to fit around the sides, filling the gaps with small bread pieces. Pour in half of the fruit mixture and cover with a slice of bread. Add the remaining fruit, cover with bread and press down securely. Make sure that there are no gaps. Press a small plate or saucer down on top and weight it with a heavy tin or a metal weight. Leave in the refrigerator for at least one day before serving.

To turn out the pudding, run the point of a thin knife carefully around the edge of the pudding to loosen it from the basin. Cover with a serving plate and invert the pudding quickly. Remove the basin and serve. You can pour more crème de cassis over the top if wished. Makes 6 servings.

Warm-up and work your upper body

This month you discover the work-out proper with a whole programme of antenatal exercises to keep you fit and strong. There are warming-up exercises, arm, back, upper body and waist trimming exercises. Make these part of your daily routine and set aside a regular time each day when you practise them. This can be first thing in the morning, during the day or before you go to bed at night – whenever is most convenient to you. They should become as natural and essential as, say, washing your face or eating.

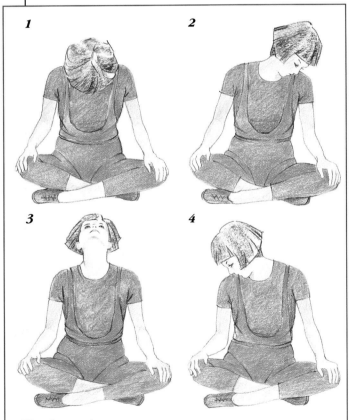

Head rotations
*1 Sit cross-legged on the floor with your hands resting lightly on your knees. Roll your head forwards with chin resting on chest.
2 Roll it to the side. 3 Then roll it round to the back as far as it will go. 4 Roll it to the other side and come full circle to the front. Repeat 3 times each way.*

Thigh toner
Sit with knees bent outwards and feet together. Pull heels in close. Lean forwards and press elbows onto knees. Hold for count of 10. Repeat 5 times.

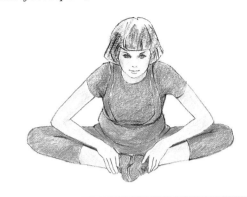

They are all designed to work specific muscle groups and areas of the body that may grow slack and weak through inactivity and prone to put on weight. Work your way through slowly and try not to miss a day. You will soon start to feel the benefits and you will feel strange if a day goes by without exercising. Remember the rules for safe exercise laid down in the previous chapter and do wear some loose clothing and put down a mat and some cushions on the floor before you start.

Warming-up
During pregnancy you will feel more sluggish than usual and it will take longer to warm-up and get your muscles moving and working. This is due in part to the increased levels of the hormones progesterone and oestrogen in your body. The warm-up has several aims:
1 To ease out stiff muscles and joints and so help prevent injury.
2 To increase circulation so that your blood can carry more oxygen to fuel your muscles.
3 To keep the joints flexible by gentle rotation.
4 To prepare you for the exercises proper.
The warm-up focuses on gentle head and shoulder rolls to ease out tension in these areas; foot and ankle rotations; and stretching out your back and legs. The angry cat pose is good for tired, aching back muscles and is borrowed from yoga. It helps take the weight of your growing abdomen off your back muscles.

All the exercises pictured here will help you to warm-up and loosen-up before you go into the pregnancy work-out proper. Practise them before

Angry cat

1 Kneel with arms and legs in line, supporting weight evenly. 2 Slowly raise your back and drop head and shoulders. Exhale. Tighten buttocks and pull in pelvic floor muscles. Inhale slowly and relax.

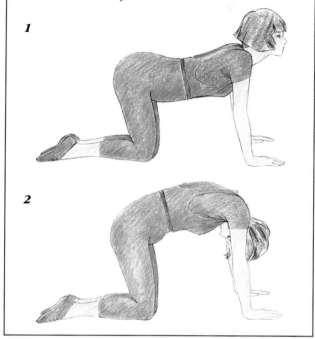

1

2

you do any exercises, whether they are floor exercises at home or at your local exercise class, or even before you go for a cycle or a swim. They will only take a few minutes so do not be tempted to skimp on them. You can perform them at other times, too. For example, when you are tired and want to relax or relieve tension in your body, especially an aching back, neck and shoulders, you can sit down quietly and do the head rotations. They are surprisingly soothing and bring instant relief.

You can also do the exercises featured in the warm-up *after* your work-out in order to cool down and relax.

All the exercises shown overleaf are for the chest, arms and waist. They will help tone up these areas

Foot rotations

1 Sit cross-legged on the floor with your back straight. Take your left knee in hands and lift foot off the floor. 2 Slowly rotate it in as large a circle as possible, pointing your toes upwards on the up movement and downwards on the down movement. 3 Take your right knee in both hands. 4 Repeat the rotation movement with right leg. Do 10 repetitions each side.

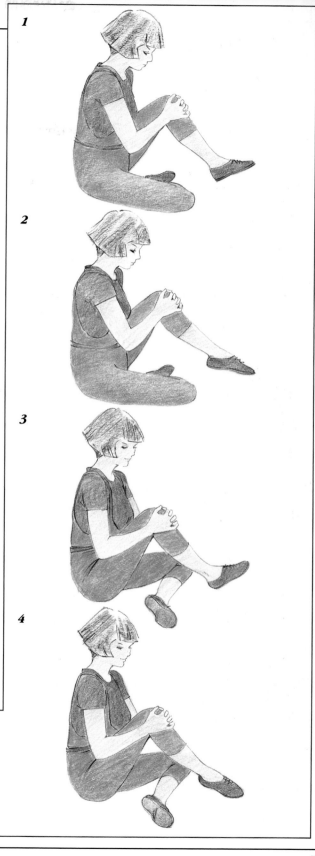

1

2

3

4

Warm-up and work your upper body

and keep them firm. You cannot stop your waistline expanding during pregnancy, but you can prevent excess fat building up in this area and keep the muscles working properly. This will help you to regain your figure more quickly after the birth of your baby, and get back into your pre-pregnancy clothes.

One of the areas that goes flabby in a lot of women is the upper arms. The wall push-ups and other arm exercises will help keep arms firm and slim. They will strengthen the muscles, too, so that you are better able to carry a heavy baby around later on, to lift her out of her cot and support her at bath-time. The arm exercises also improve the general circulation in your upper body and strengthen the muscles that support your breasts, which will inevitably get larger and heavier as the weeks pass. Although a well-fitting support bra is essential, these exercises will help work the muscles underneath the breasts to help you retain their natural shape. Heavy, sagging breasts and your enlarged uterus can pull you forwards and affect your upright posture, putting more strain on back muscles and causing or exacerbating backache.

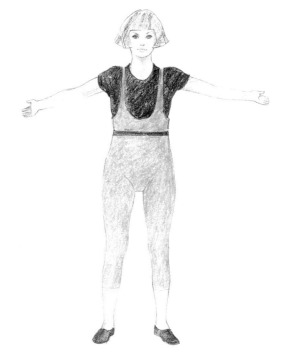

Upper arm toners
1 Stand with your feet hip distance apart, crossing arms at shoulder level across the upper chest. 2 Take a deep breath and throw open your arms as wide as they will go. Exhale and cross them again. Repeat the exercise 20 times. This will help strengthen your upper arm muscles.

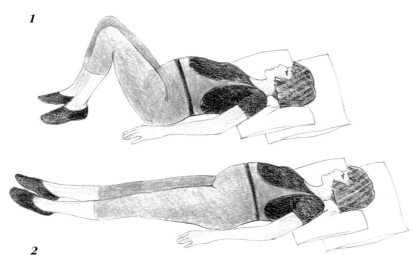

Leg sliding
1 Lie on the floor on your back with some cushions to support your head and shoulders, knees bent, and press the small of your back into the floor. 2 Gently slide your legs down to the floor. Now keeping your back flat on the floor, raise one knee and then the other. Repeat 10 times. Stretch slowly and gradually and always stop if you feel uncomfortable.

If you cannot do the exercises easily at first and find the stretching difficult, do not worry nor try to overdo it. Just take them slowly and gradually – you will get stronger and more flexible with practice. Maintain your posture throughout and only stretch as far as feels comfortable. If a stretch becomes painful, stop immediately and rest before you attempt another exercise. In particular, do not try anything that puts strain on your uterus and makes this area feel painful.

It cannot be repeated too often how important it is to build a programme of antenatal exercises such as these into your daily routine if you are to avoid gaining excessive weight and to get your pre-pregnancy figure back afterwards. It is always easy to find excuses not to exercise, especially if you are busy with a full-time job or a young family, but the far-reaching benefits of regular exercise make all the effort worthwhile. What's more, you will start enjoying these sessions and will miss them if you skip a day. Also, you will feel decidedly fitter and stronger and with this comes a greater sense of well-being and a new awareness of your own body.

Some women have said that they did not really

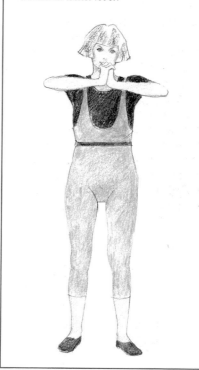

Bust shaper

Stand feet hip distance apart, arms at shoulder level. Clasp one fist in the other and press hands together. Hold for 10 and relax. Repeat at bust and waist level.

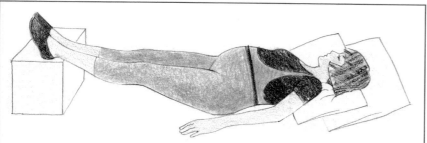

Bridging

1 Lie flat on the floor with some cushions to support your head and shoulders, arms at your side and your feet raised and resting on a low box or stool.

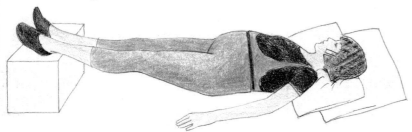

2 Pull in and tighten your buttocks and pelvic floor muscles and, keeping your back straight, slowly lift your buttocks and lower back off the floor. Hold for a count of 10 and then relax and slowly lower your buttocks. Repeat 10 times. This is good for the pelvic floor, abdominal and buttock muscles and improves circulation in the legs. Also you will find it an easy and gentle exercise to do and you can gradually build up the number of repetitions when you feel ready.

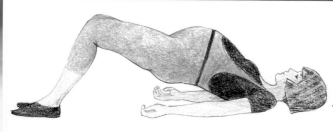

Buttocks squeezing

1 Lie on your back with your feet flat on the floor hip distance apart and knees bent. 2 With your arms at your sides, palms facing upwards, gently raise your hips off the floor and gradually squeeze your buttocks tightly together, followed by your pelvic floor muscles. 3 Hold for a few seconds and then slowly release the pelvic floor muscles as you lower yourself to the floor. Repeat 4 times.

Warm-up and work your upper body

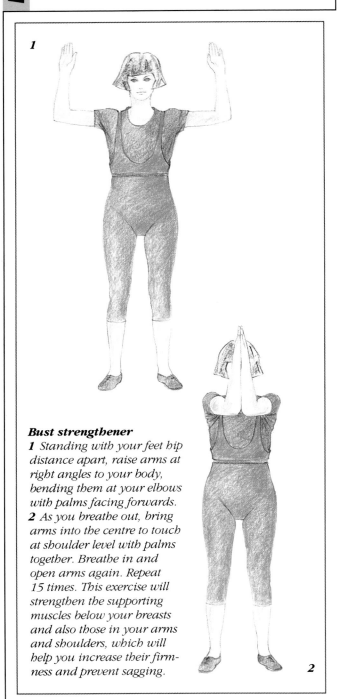

Bust strengthener
1 Standing with your feet hip distance apart, raise arms at right angles to your body, bending them at your elbows with palms facing forwards.
2 As you breathe out, bring arms into the centre to touch at shoulder level with palms together. Breathe in and open arms again. Repeat 15 times. This exercise will strengthen the supporting muscles below your breasts and also those in your arms and shoulders, which will help you increase their firmness and prevent sagging.

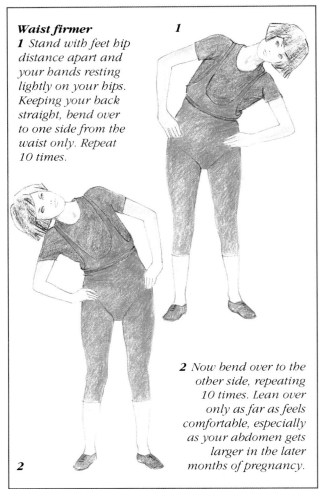

Waist firmer
1 Stand with feet hip distance apart and your hands resting lightly on your hips. Keeping your back straight, bend over to one side from the waist only. Repeat 10 times.

2 Now bend over to the other side, repeating 10 times. Lean over only as far as feels comfortable, especially as your abdomen gets larger in the later months of pregnancy.

know themselves and how their bodies functioned until they started exercising during pregnancy. This is a time in your life when your mind tends to be focused inwards on the changes taking place in your body and the new life growing within you. Listen to your body as you exercise – get to know its limitations and its strengths. Treat it with respect and never demand impossible feats from it. You will be surprised to discover how it works and its capabilities.

But do remember that pregnancy is not the right time for testing your body out and asking it to surmount new goals. Always stretch and exercise with care, even in these early months before your bump starts to show and you still feel relatively slim. Over-exercising can not only strain or tear muscles and cause you to feel tired – it can also be potentially harmful to your baby if you exercise *too* much for *too* long and put *too* much strain on your back and abdominal muscles.

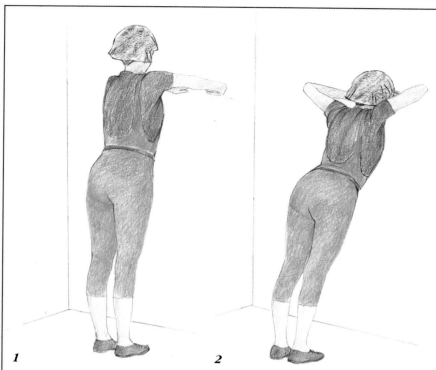

Wall push-ups

1 Stand with your feet hip distance apart, facing a wall. Rest your hands at shoulder level on the wall, palms down and facing inwards. **2** Slowly lower your body towards the wall until your elbows bend and your nose is touching the wall. Gradually straighten your arms and raise your body back to the starting position. Repeat 15 times. Make sure that your feet stay flat on the ground throughout and exhale deeply as you raise your body, inhaling as you lower it towards the wall. This is an excellent exercise for keeping your breasts firm and in shape.

1

2

Waist toner

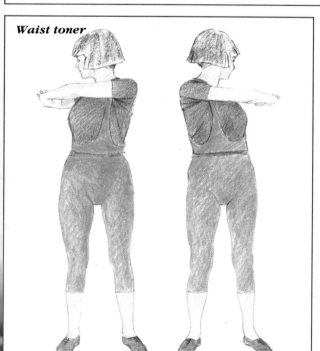

1 Stand with feet apart. Bend elbows at shoulder level, holding one fist inside your other hand. Swivel your upper body round from the waist and inhale deeply. Repeat 10 times. **2** Exhale and do same on other side.

Waist stretches

1 Standing with your feet hip distance apart, your left foot turned slightly outwards and your right foot inwards, raise your arms and extend them at shoulder level straight out on either side. Slowly bend over towards your out-stretched left foot until your hand touches it. Hold your right arm straight up above you. **2** Gently raise yourself up and repeat to the right side. Do 3 repetitions.

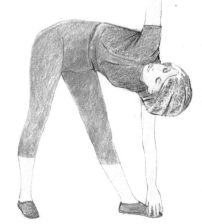

Gain weight sensibly with fibre foods

You

By now you should be looking radiant, healthy and 'blooming' and really enjoying your pregnancy. You may have to start wearing specially designed maternity clothes this month, but don't spend a fortune on them – there are some very reasonably priced ones in specialist stores. If you are dismayed to find that you are putting on weight on your hips, thighs and bottom as well as at the front, now is the time to start your pregnancy work-out and perform it religiously every day. These fatty pads are inevitable to some extent as your body lays down reserves for breast-feeding. They will gradually disappear in the year following the birth of your baby. However, regular exercise will help strengthen your muscles in preparation for the delivery and for supporting the growing weight of the baby in the months to come. It will also prevent you putting on excessive weight in unwanted areas. By the end of the fifth month your weight may be nearly 7kg/14lb above normal, although this obviously varies depending on your physical make-up, diet and metabolism.

You will now be very aware of the baby moving inside you. Sometimes she will be very active indeed, while at others she may seem to be asleep. Unfortunately you will probably feel her most when you are sitting down resting in the evenings or when you lie down in bed at night. It is easier for the baby to move when you are lying down or sitting comfortably with your feet up. When you are moving around, you tend to rock her in your pelvis and this probably helps her to fall asleep.

If you are experiencing difficulties sleeping or feel uncomfortable and awkward in bed with your growing 'bump' getting in the way, you would

Eat plenty of fibre-rich foods

To avoid constipation which is a common problem for many women in pregnancy, make sure that you include plenty of fibre in your diet. Good sources are daily helpings of vegetables, fresh fruit, whole-grain cereals such as muesli, brown rice, 100 per cent wholemeal bread, and bran sprinkled over your breakfast cereal or dessert. Fibre is the indigestible part of plants which provides roughage and bulk in the diet. It keeps our bowels healthy and working regularly. It also helps dilute and expel any toxic substances in our bodies so it is especially beneficial in pregnancy to help prevent straining which may lead to varicose veins and piles.

High fibre	Good fibre	Low fibre
bran	banana	tomatoes
beans	avocado	mashed potatoes
baked potato	celery	white bread
wholemeal bread	nuts	lettuce
prunes	carrots	white pasta
dried fruit	apples	white rice
brown rice	oranges	white flour
peas, sweetcorn	pineapple	plums
leafy green vegetables	figs	cherries
pears	grapefruit	radishes
strawberries	cauliflower	pumpkin, squash
broccoli	beetroot	cucumber
lentils	celery	watercress
Bran Flakes	pearl barley	grapes
All Bran	aubergine	damsons
raspberries	mango	beansprouts
Weetabix		asparagus

be well advised now to support your tummy with a cushion or pillow. Lie on your side with a pillow under your 'bump' and perhaps another one positioned strategically underneath your outstretched knee. Most women find this position for sleeping very comfortable.

This month, you might experience your first bout of heartburn – one of the most annoying problems in pregnancy. To try and avoid it as much as possible, don't eat too late or go to bed on top of your meal. Eat early and sit up straight to rest afterwards so that the upper part of the uterus is not pressing on the stomach and thus causing food mixed with gastric juices to be pushed back up into your oesophagus. Eating smaller meals more regularly and avoiding spicy, fried foods can also help. Stick to plain, simple food made with natural, wholesome ingredients. If you do get an attack of heartburn, deal with it naturally rather than taking an antacid preparation. Sipping a glass of milk slowly often helps. Too many antacid mixtures are potentially harmful to your baby, and bicarbonate of soda/baking soda destroys valuable B-vitamins in your body which your baby needs for her healthy development.

The top of your uterus will soon reach the level of your navel and you will notice that your abdomen is getting progressively rounder. At the same time, your breasts will be getting rounder and fuller, too, in preparation for breast-feeding. If you haven't already bought a support bra, do so now. It will make you feel more comfortable and help preserve the firm shape of your breasts and prevent them flopping after the birth.

If you have a family history of varicose veins, or any warning signals of broken veins showing on your legs, make sure that you put your feet up level with the rest of your body as often as possible. Regular exercise such as walking, swimming or cycling will improve circulation in the lower half of your body and relieve congestion in the valves, as will foot rotations (*see* page 73). Don't wear tight, restricting clothes, cross your legs when you sit down or allow yourself to become constipated. These are all contributory factors. A healthy diet that is rich in fibre and vitamin E helps prevent varicose veins forming.

Your baby

By the end of this month your baby will be about 25cm/10in long and will weigh 450g/1lb. She will also have developed what is known as the *vernix caseosa* – a creamy protective covering that stops the skin becoming waterlogged. If you could see her face now, it would still look a little strange as her eyes are closed and bulging because the skin around them has not yet plumped out.

Her lungs are developing in preparation for her entry into the world when she will need them for breathing. However, in the darkness and safety of the uterus she receives all the oxygen she needs via the placenta. It flows directly into her own circulatory system and the deoxygenated blood is then carried away by the placenta. The baby is still growing rapidly in weight and length and her muscles are developing and getting stronger. This accounts for why her movements are becoming more noticeable and why you can feel her little feet kicking you. There is still plenty of room for her to move about inside the amniotic sac in which she is suspended in fluid, and where she can twist and kick freely.

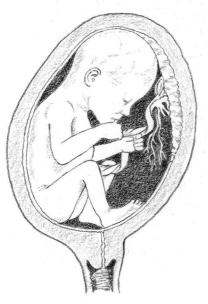

Your baby's face is now almost fully formed and she even has tiny toenails. You will feel her moving about and even kicking you. Her legs are now in proportion to her body size.

Healthy, white teeth for a confident smile

You can smile with confidence throughout your pregnancy if your teeth are gleaming white and healthy. This is an important time for practising good dental hygiene. In early pregnancy the gums soften and the veins in them enlarge. They are more easily damaged and infected than usual and this can trigger off decay. The extra acid in your mouth puts your teeth at risk, too, and the baby makes additional demands on your calcium supplies – so important for maintaining strong, healthy teeth.

There is an old saying that you will lose a tooth for every child you bear. Don't let this come true for you. Look after your teeth and they won't let you down. A sympathetic dentist and daily oral hygiene can help prevent tooth decay and bleeding gums. As usual it is your hormonal balance that is causing all the problems – the increased oestrogen in your body causes gums to swell somewhat. It varies for different women, but eating a really healthy wholefoods diet which supplies all the essential nutrients, and regular flossing will both help.

Visiting the dentist

You should visit your dentist early on in your pregnancy for a check-up and in order to have your teeth professionally cleaned and scaled to remove any build-up of yellowish tartar. You will be amazed at how white and clean they look afterwards. This is not at all painful and a great beauty treatment. Tell the dentist that you are pregnant and do not want an X-ray. Although your mouth is a long way away from your abdomen, you should *never* be exposed to X-rays in early pregnancy as they may cause damage to your unborn child. Nor should you have gas if you need an extraction – it may cross the placenta into the baby. Most local injections are OK but you should check with your doctor or dentist first just to be on the safe side.

Tooth decay

The biggest cause of modern tooth decay is sugar

and you should definitely cut down your intake to a minimum during pregnancy while your teeth and gums are very susceptible. Sugar contributes to a build-up of plaque on the teeth and gums – a mixture of bacteria, saliva and food residue which adheres to the teeth and settles in the cracks between them and round the gumline to eventually cause decay and gum disease. Look in the mirror at your teeth. They may well look healthy, clean, white and shining but do not be deceived – plaque is lurking there, invisible and colourless. You can prove this very simply by carrying out a test with a disclosing tablet – available from good drugstores and chemists. Brush your teeth as usual. They will feel clean and your mouth will seem fresh and sweet-tasting, but normal brushing usually misses out on up to 80 per cent of the plaque in your mouth. Now dissolve a disclosing tablet in your mouth and look again in the mirror – the areas of plaque which the toothbrush has missed will show up as bright alarming red or purple. There's a lot, isn't there?

Plaque settles around the necks of the teeth and in the spaces between them. It damages them in two ways: it leads to the formation of hard, yellowish tartar that requires professional scaling to remove it; and it produces acids that attack the enamel of the teeth and start the long, slow process of the decay.

Brushing

You should brush your teeth at least twice a day, first thing in the morning and last thing at night. Better still is to brush after every meal to help remove food particles that may lead to plaque. This will help keep teeth strong and gums healthy. Choose a soft or medium toothbrush with thin rounded bristles – a bristle brush is preferable to nylon. Remember that a toothbrush does not last for ever and it should be replaced once every three months for the sake of hygiene and wear and tear. It may need replacement earlier still if the bristles start to bend and become misshapen. After brushing always hang your brush, head up to dry, after rinsing out thoroughly under a cold running tap. You can buy special toothbrush holders attached to the wall by screws or suction caps very cheaply for this purpose. Never stand your brush in a glass with other brushes.

Look after your teeth during pregnancy so that you can keep your healthy smile without fillings.

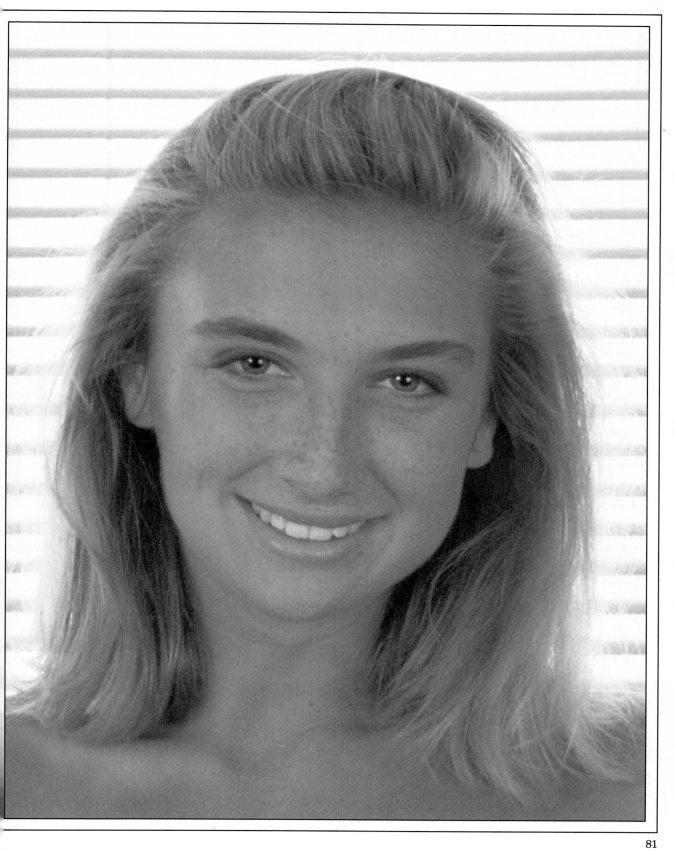

Healthy, white teeth for a confident smile

Many dentists recommend using a toothpaste containing fluoride to preserve healthy teeth and gums. When you brush, make sure that you brush in the direction in which the tooth grows *away* from the gums. Holding the brush at an angle of 45°, start at the back of your mouth and work round the sides to the front teeth. Be sure to brush the backs of the teeth as well as the fronts that show. Rinse your mouth out thoroughly afterwards to remove all traces of toothpaste, and then floss as described next.

Flossing

You should make flossing a daily part of your beauty regime. After a while it will become instinctive to floss after brushing. This will help control the build-up of harmful bacteria in your mouth and reduce the risk of tooth decay and gum disease. Choose the unwaxed type of dental floss and break off a length of about 45cm/18in. Wind the ends round the index fingers of each hand leaving a free section in the middle. Now, keeping it taut, work it backwards and forwards between the teeth in a gentle sawing action. Coax it gently into the crevices around the gums but take care not to be brutal and make your gums bleed, although this may happen initially however careful you are until your teeth get used to it. Practised regularly, flossing will help remove plaque effectively and is well worth the effort.

Diet and your teeth

Although the major cause of tooth decay is sugar, deficiencies of important nutrients can also contribute to disease and decay. Teeth are composed of the hardest substance in the human body – calcium phosphate – and they need calcium in order to be strong and healthy. You can obtain calcium from milk, yoghurt, cheese, eggs, leafy green vegetables and sardines. However, in order for the calcium to be absorbed and used by your body you also need adequate vitamin D. Luckily for you this vitamin tends to be found in foods that contain a high degree of calcium too so you should be able to get both at the same time – for example, in milk, eggs, cheese and butter. The best sources, however, are fish liver oils, sardines, herring, mackerel, salmon, tuna and most oily fish. You should be careful not to overdo your vitamin D intake. It can be toxic and potentially harmful to both your health and that of your baby if taken in excessive doses as it is fat-soluble and stored by the body. You do *not* need to take a supplement. It is better to eat sensibly.

You will also need vitamins B6 and C to build up your gums' resistance to infection and prevent bleeding. Your wholefoods diet of whole-grain cereals, offal, citrus fruits, potatoes and brewers yeast will supply these nutrients. Vitamin C is especially important as it strengthens the connective tissue.

It is also worth knowing that the quality of your diet during pregnancy can affect the future teeth of

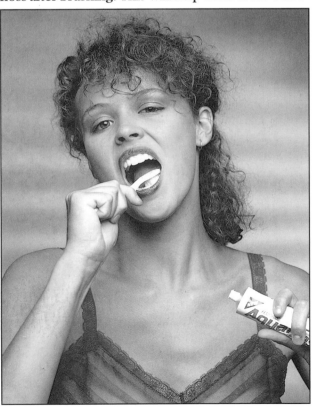

Daily flossing and brushing will help prevent the build-up of potentially damaging plaque on your teeth and gums. Wind some dental floss around your index fingers and move it backwards and forwards between your teeth.

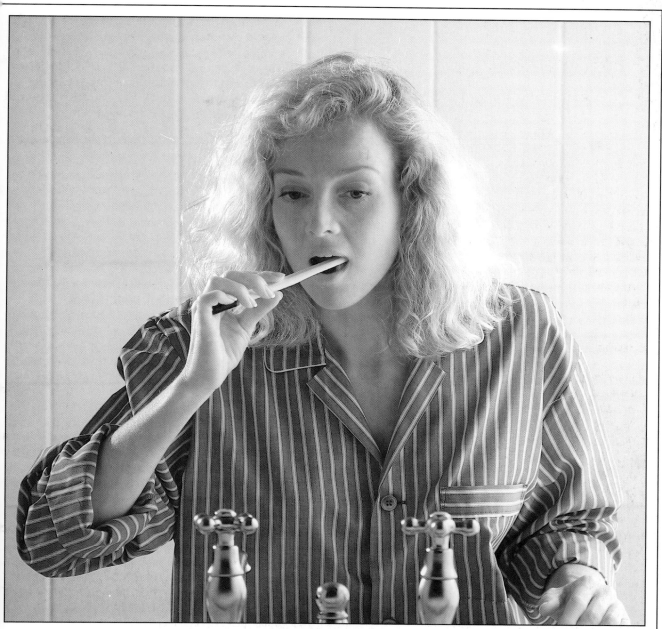

your baby as well as your own. The size and quality of her teeth, the shape of her jaw at birth and their susceptibility to decay are all determined to some extent by your intake of calcium and other vital nutrients. An inadequate calcium intake may cause your child to have overcrowded, crooked or poorly formed teeth later on in life. Thus it is important to maintain the quality of your diet during breastfeeding and wean your baby onto healthy foods.

There is a lot to be said for the old adage that an apple a day keeps the doctor away – or at least as far as your teeth are concerned. Apples, celery and carrots all clean and strengthen teeth. They also make good, low-calorie snacks when you are pregnant. Because you have to chew them hard, they tend to fill you up better than crisps and other unhealthy foods. Be sure to avoid sugary snacks such as chocolate, sweets, cakes, pastries and buns. It must be stressed that sugar is the worst enemy of your teeth, together with white flour. So if you have a very sweet tooth, you must make strenuous efforts to curb it, or to find healthier alternatives such as fresh fruit.

Quality not quantity – eating for two

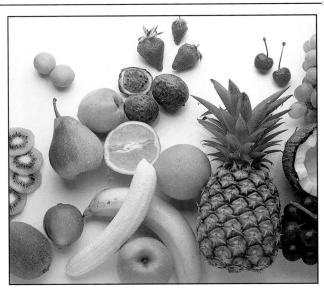

Many women who become pregnant worry needlessly about gaining weight and how they will ever recover their figures after the baby is born. Some are so concerned about this that they actually try to slim while they are pregnant. It cannot be emphasized enough how dangerous this can be. When you are pregnant you need *extra*, not *less*, calories in order to stay fit and well and to have a healthy baby.

This does not mean that eating for two implies eating enough for two people and helping yourself to double portions of food. However, it does mean that you have to improve the quality of what you eat. It has been estimated that during the first three months of pregnancy you will need an additional 150 calories daily – this equates to approximately two extra slices of very thinly buttered wholemeal bread. And during the next six months you will need 350 extra calories every day – approximately the same as 50g/2oz salted nuts. So you can see that you need not eat enormous amounts of extra food.

The important thing is to concentrate on high-quality, nutrient-rich food which is often low to medium in calories. Avoid the low-quality, high-calorie foods that put on unwanted weight and have little or no nutritional goodness – for example, cakes, candies, sweets, buns, cream, pastries, sugar, biscuits and chocolates. You will get all the calories and nutrients you need from eating less fattening fresh vegetables, fruit, whole-grain cereals, lean meat, fish, poultry, beans, pulses, milk, eggs and low- to medium-fat cheeses and yoghurts.

Restricting your weight gain

In the past many doctors encouraged women to restrict their weight gain deliberately and to eat less than usual. This was because they believed that a high weight gain may be linked with toxaemia, a term that embraces those disorders in later pregnancy where there is increased fluid, swelling and high blood pressure. However, new scientific research shows that the women most likely to become toxaemic are those on poor diets which are high in processed foods and low in nutrients, and those who try to restrict their weight gain.

These women are more inclined to have low-birth-weight babies, to have longer, more difficult labours and to suffer haemorrhages. Even their babies may be at risk and have a bigger chance of being retarded or handicapped in some way, or having a lower IQ score in later childhood.

If you restrict your own weight gain, you are more likely to have a smaller baby. After all, your baby can only get the food and nutrients she needs to grow and develop that you provide. Babies weighing in at 7lb or more are generally healthier, stronger and even more intelligent than smaller babies, especially those of 5½lb or less.

The average weight gain during the whole of pregnancy is about 28lb. Mothers who put on this much weight and eat a healthy, nutritious diet tend to have bigger, healthier babies and fewer complications. Usually the baby's weight increases proportionately to the mother's weight gain. If you breastfeed your baby afterwards and do the postnatal exercises regularly you will soon regain your figure and normal weight without any

	Weight gain in lbs
Baby's birth weight	7½
Enlarged uterus	2
Placenta	1½
Amniotic fluid	2
Enlarged breasts	1½
Increased blood volume	4
Increased body fluids and fat	9½
Total weight gain	28lb

problems. To show you how the extra weight is all accounted for, look at the chart.

You can see that only one-third of the total weight gain is actually accounted for by a increase in fat and fluid in your own body. The rest belongs to the baby and its life support system which you will shed anyway at birth; your enlarged breasts which will reduce after breastfeeding; increased blood volume will gradually be discounted after birth as will the enlarged uterus.

This example is obviously only an approximation, and weight gain and how it is made up will vary from one woman to the next. Fluid retention in particular may account for a large gain in some women. Don't be alarmed if this happens to you – it usually disappears soon after delivery.

Of course, the ideal amount of gain will also be influenced by your pre-pregnancy weight. If you are underweight at the time of conception, it may be beneficial if you gain quite a lot of weight while eating a highly nutritious pregnancy diet. On the other hand, if you are very overweight when you become pregnant you may not need to gain so much weight as long as your baby receives all the nutrients that are vital for her growth and development.

The best thing is just to eat a healthy, varied diet which does not contain too many high-fat, sugared and convenience foods. Regular antenatal exercises, walking and swimming will help tone up and firm muscles and problem areas and prevent superfluous weight gain. One way of checking whether you are gaining too much weight in unwanted places is to measure your upper thighs. This thigh measurement should stay roughly the same throughout your pregnancy.

How much and when?
Well, many doctors think that a pregnant woman should gain about 10lb in the first 20 weeks, and then a steady weight gain of about 1lb per week for the next 20 weeks up to birth, making a total of about 30lb. Of course, not everyone conforms to this perfect norm and you should not be unduly worried if your weight fluctuates a little and you gain more one week than you do another. You may even find that some weeks you don't gain any at all. You will be weighed whenever you visit the doctor or clinic and they will check that everything is OK and that there is nothing to worry about.

Should you watch the calories?
Pregnancy is not a time for counting calories and restricting your weight as already mentioned. However, although some weight gain of, say 28-35lb is healthy, it is not a good idea for your health or your looks to put on excessive weight. High-calorie foods that provide little nutritional goodness should be cut out altogether or eaten only as occasional treats – for example, biscuits, cookies, chocolate, sweets, cream, steamed puddings, cakes, buns, doughnuts and the like. Remember, too, that some savoury foods can be very fattening and aren't particularly good for you – French fries, potato crisps, processed sausages and most fried foods. Always grill meat and fish in preference to frying them – the calorie count will be lower and the end-

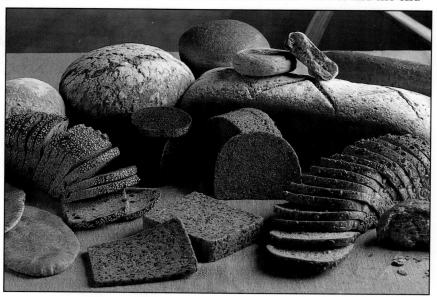

Eating healthily can be easy and fun. Fruit is full of vitamins and minerals so try some of the different kinds available in shops and markets. For a change follow some of these recipes, using fruit in nutritious and tasty, but low-calorie, puddings. It is also easy to vary your fibre intake as there is a wide range of different breads, rolls and cereals to choose from. However, try to select bread that has not been baked with additititves.

Quality not quantity – eating for two

product healthier. Here are some recipes for enjoyable cakes and desserts, which are nutritious and really do you good. Although some efforts have been made to restrict calories, they should not be eaten in large quantities and should be regarded as treats rather than everyday fare. The healthiest dessert you can eat is fresh fruit or yoghurt; and the best snacks are raw vegetables, nuts and seeds. However, if you have a naturally sweet tooth, the recipes here may help make your pregnancy diet more bearable.

Teatime

If you usually eat afternoon tea, make it as healthy and nutritious as possible. Wholemeal sandwiches filled with salad stuff, cottage cheese, peanut butter, apple and pear spread or marmite provide fibre, vitamins and minerals as well as protein. Wholemeal muffins can be split, toasted and thinly buttered in winter. Cheese, celery sticks and a bowl of watercress will add a savoury flavour as will hard-boiled eggs. Instead of chocolate cake, make an easy fruit cake with wholemeal flour and less sugar, or some delicious wholemeal squares or slices filled with dried apricots or dates. Zucchini nut loaf may sound odd but it is a fantastic teabread sliced and buttered. There are so many wholefood recipes to try, and they are easy to make in a food processor or food mixer. Take shortcuts whenever you can to save time and labour. If you are still working or busy with young children, you could cook in bulk when you have some spare time and freeze several cakes or loaves until needed.

Zucchini nut loaf

3 eggs
175g/6oz/³⁄4 cup soft brown sugar
100ml/4floz/¹⁄2 cup oil (preferably walnut)
150g/5oz/1¹⁄4 cups wholemeal flour
150g/5oz/1¹⁄4 cups plain flour
5ml/1 teaspoon baking powder
2.5ml/¹⁄2 teaspoon bicarbonate of soda

5ml/1 teaspoon cinnamon
2.5ml/¹⁄2 teaspoon each allspice and ginger
pinch of salt
2 courgettes/zucchini, finely grated
50g/2oz/¹⁄3 cup chopped dates
50g/2oz/¹⁄2 cup chopped hazelnuts

Beat the eggs, sugar and oil until well-blended or process in a food processor. Gently stir in the sifted flours, baking powder, bicarbonate of soda, spices and salt. Fold in the grated courgette/zucchini, the dates and hazelnuts. Pour into a greased, lined loaf tin and bake in a preheated oven at 180°C, 350°F, gas 4 for 1 hour 20 minutes, or until the loaf is well-risen and cooked. Cool, slice and butter.

Crunchy granola bars

25g/1oz/¹⁄4 cup flaked almonds, chopped
25g/1oz/¹⁄4 cup shelled hazelnuts, chopped
75g/3oz/¹⁄2 cup California raisins
50g/2oz/¹⁄4 cup soft brown sugar
100g/4oz/1¹⁄3 cups porridge oats
25g/1oz sesame seeds
60ml/4 tablespoons sunflower oil
60ml/4 tablespoons honey

Grease a shallow oblong 18 × 28cm/7 × 11in tin, and mix together all the ingredients in a bowl until thoroughly blended. Press the mixture lightly into the prepared tin and bake at 180°C, 350°F, gas 4 for 25 minutes until light golden. Cool in the tin for 5 minutes, then mark into squares with a sharp knife. Cool for a further 10 minutes, then remove to a cooling rack. Makes 8 squares.

Avocado harvest teabread

225g/8oz/2¹⁄4 cups self-raising flour
1.25ml/¹⁄4 teaspoon bicarbonate of soda
2.5ml/¹⁄2 teaspoon salt
2.5ml/¹⁄2 teaspoon cinnamon
75g/3oz/³⁄4 cup butter
350g/12oz mashed avocado flesh
175g/6oz/³⁄4 cup sugar
2 eggs, beaten
100g/4oz/²⁄3 cup raisins

Grease and line a 1kg/2lb loaf tin (approx. 20 × 10cm/8 × 4in). Mix the flour, bicarbonate of soda, salt and cinnamon. Cream the butter and avocado with the sugar until pale and creamy. Add the egg, a little at a time, with a little flour to prevent curdling. Beat well between each addition. Fold in the remaining flour and raisins, and place the mixture in the prepared tin.

Bake at 180°C, 350°F, gas 4 in a preheated oven for approximately 1¼ hours, or until well risen and firm. Turn out and cool on a wire rack, and serve sliced and buttered. Makes 16 slices.

Pineapple carrot cake

175g/6oz/¾ cup margarine
175g/6oz/¾ cup muscovado sugar
4 eggs
grated rind of 1 orange
225g/8oz/2¼ cups wholemeal flour
10ml/2 teaspoons each baking powder and cinnamon
150g/5oz grated carrot
150g/5oz/1 cup crushed pineapple (canned or fresh)
50g/2oz/½ cup chopped walnuts
juice of 1 large orange
Cheese and fruit frosting:
175g/6oz/1 cup curd cheese
50g/2oz/⅓ cup puréed fruit
grated rind of 1 orange
30ml/2 tablespoons icing sugar
pineapple chunks or orange segments to decorate

Cream the fat and sugar until fluffy. Beat in the eggs, one at a time. Fold in the remaining cake ingredients. If the mixture is too stiff, add a little more pineapple or orange juice. Pour into two 17.5cm/7in sandwich tins. Bake low down in a preheated oven at 180°C, 350°F, gas 4 for 45 minutes or until cooked. Cool on wire racks.

Beat all the frosting ingredients together. Fill the sponges with the mixture, sandwich together and coat the top. Decorate with fruit.

Tempting desserts
You do not have to make sacrifices and totally forego puddings just because you are pregnant – you just have to be selective and avoid the processed shop-bought ones and home-made creamy sort in favour of more nutritious dishes made with wholemeal flour or pasta, rice, honey, fresh fruit, milk, yoghurt and spices. We have concocted a few for you to try.

Fruit brochettes

225g/8oz strawberries
1 papaya, peeled and cubed
4 kumquats (or 1 banana cut in chunks and sprinkled with lemon juice)
Strawberry dip:
100g/4oz ripe strawberries
225g/8oz/1⅓ cups strawberry roulé cheese

Prepare the fruit and arrange alternately on 4 thin bamboo skewers, reserving 4 strawberries for decoration. Make the sauce: put the strawberries and roulé cheese in a blender or food processor and blend until smooth. Place a brochette and a good dollop of sauce on each of 4 plates and decorate with the reserved strawberries.

Apricot fromage frais dessert

225g/8oz/1½ cups dried apricots, soaked overnight
225g/8oz/1 cup fromage frais low-fat soft cheese
15ml/1 tablespoon honey
45ml/3 tablespoons toasted almonds or granola

Cook the apricots in the soaking water until tender and leave to cool. Drain away any excess juice and place the apricots in a liquidizer or processor with the fromage frais. Blend on high speed until thoroughly mixed and smooth. Sweeten to taste with honey. Pour into a serving dish and sprinkle with toasted almonds or granola. Makes 2-3 servings.

Fresh fruit ice-cream

225g/8oz puréed fresh fruit, eg. strawberries, raspberries, peaches, apricots, mangoes
500ml/1 pint/2½ cups milk
3 eggs, beaten
30ml/2 tablespoons clear honey
10ml/2 teaspoons lemon juice

Purée the fruit. Heat the milk, and whisk in the eggs, off the heat. Add the honey and pour into the top of a double boiler. Heat gently, stirring continuously until the mixture starts to thicken and coats the back of a spoon. Remove from the heat and cool. Beat in the puréed fruit and lemon juice. Pour into a freezing tray. Freeze for 1 hour, remove and stir. Then freeze until completely frozen. Makes 4-6 servings.

Keep your legs looking good in pregnancy

All the exercises this month are for working your leg muscles. These are very important as they have to take the extra weight of your enlarged uterus and breasts, the baby and your increased body fluids and blood volume. This, of course, makes them vulnerable to poor circulation and consequently cramping varicose veins. Regular exercises will strengthen the muscles in your legs so that they tire less easily. They will increase circulation and the stimulated blood flow will reduce the likelihood of cramps and the formation of varicose veins.

Most women do not have a hint of varicose veins until they become pregnant but they can be prevented even then if you exercise regularly and eat plenty of high-fibre foods. They usually appear when some prolonged obstruction to the flow of blood in the veins of the legs back to the heart raises the pressure inside the veins. In time, this causes them to dilate. About 90 per cent of the blood from your feet and lower legs returns to the heart through one big vein in the groin. If this vein becomes blocked and compressed, usually in the pelvis, then the blood has to find alternative routes through the small veins near the surface of your legs. Although they were previously invisible, this causes them to become distended and swollen and the end result is usually unwanted ugly varicose veins.

Regular exercise encourages better circulation in the legs and feet and relieves congestion in the valves. The stretching exercises shown here are most beneficial as are walking, swimming and cycling. Even when you are sitting down in the office, talking to friends or watching television, you can practise some foot rotations (see page 73). If you are standing waiting for a train or bus, move your legs about and shift from foot to foot. This will boost sluggish circulation and prevent the pooling of the blood. Never sit with your legs crossed as this too inhibits circulation, and try to put your legs and feet up at least once a day for more than 30 minutes. Another good passive exercise to introduce into your daily routine for avoiding varicose veins is to lie on the floor, your head and shoulders supported by cushions and your feet raised above you and resting

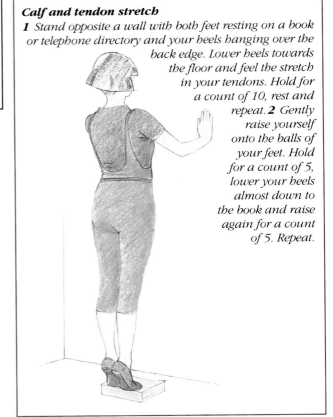

Calf and tendon stretch
1 Stand opposite a wall with both feet resting on a book or telephone directory and your heels hanging over the back edge. Lower heels towards the floor and feel the stretch in your tendons. Hold for a count of 10, rest and repeat. 2 Gently raise yourself onto the balls of your feet. Hold for a count of 5, lower your heels almost down to the book and raise again for a count of 5. Repeat.

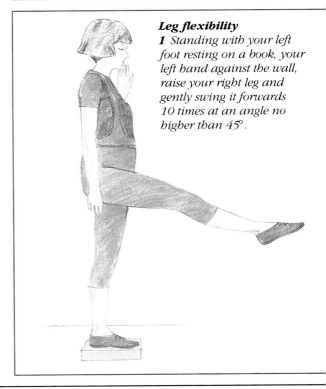

Leg flexibility
1 Standing with your left foot resting on a book, your left hand against the wall, raise your right leg and gently swing it forwards 10 times at an angle no higher than 45°.

Calf stretch

1 Stand facing a wall, your palms resting lightly on it. Rise up onto the balls of your feet.

2 With knees bent, gently lower your heels almost down to the floor and then rise up again on your toes. Do 20 repetitions.

3 Move left leg forwards and bend knees. With feet flat on floor, stretch right leg behind. Lift right heel and press down. Repeat with other leg.

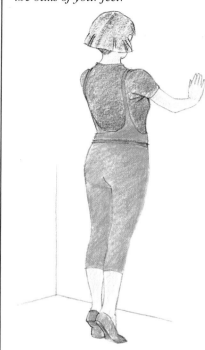 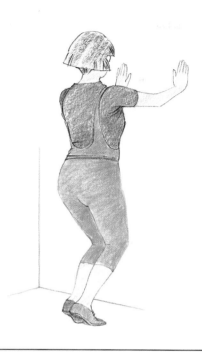 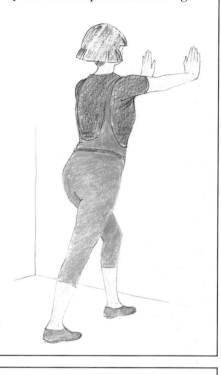

2 With your left foot still flat on the book, slowly swing your right leg backwards 10 times. Do not raise your leg too high in the air.

3 Next swing your right leg out to the side, once again not lifting it too far off the ground. Do 10 repetitions.

4 Swing your leg backwards and outwards at an angle of not more than 45°. Do this 10 times then repeat all four movements with the other leg.

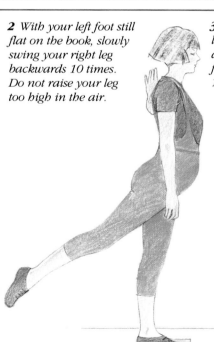 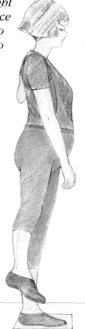 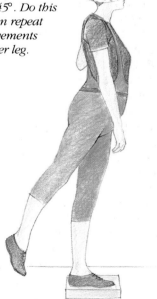

Keep your legs looking good in pregnancy

on a wall. Practise your pelvic floor exercises while you lie there and hold the position for about 10 minutes. You will feel remarkably refreshed and relaxed afterwards.

Of course, a healthy diet that is high in fibre will also help prevent varicose veins. If you are following the guidelines laid down for eating in pregnancy at the beginning of the book, you will minimize the likelihood of getting varicose veins.

Other leg problems during pregnancy

Regular exercise can help prevent other problems with your legs including cramping, tired, aching muscles and swelling in the area. Wearing flat, comfortable shoes, not high heels, will help exercise your leg muscles more efficiently, improve your posture and avoid swollen feet and ankles. Any exercise will increase circulation and, surprising though it may seem, minimize instances of aching legs. Standing still for too long in one place is more tiring to your legs and feet than being on the move. Swimming is particularly beneficial as it exercises your legs and gives them a thorough work-out in a near-weightless state without your legs having to support your body.

Whenever you can at home, remove your shoes and walk barefoot. This has the dual advantages of helping to prevent swelling from tight shoes and heat, and strengthens your feet and ankles, too. The best exercise of all for your legs is pure and simple walking, so walk whenever you can, whether you live in a big city or in the country. Practise breathing deeply and fully as you walk and be aware of your posture (see pages 124-7). Make sure, above all, your feet are comfortable and that your shoes support you properly and do not rub or pinch your feet. You will enjoy walking if you feel relaxed and without any discomfort. This is one of the most enjoyable times of your pregnancy when you are beginning to blossom and your bump is getting ever larger but not yet cumbersome. In the months to come, as it gets bigger it may feel heavy and you may even experience unfamiliar sensations in the pelvic floor area as the baby presses down as you walk. If these

become stronger and quite painful, you should stop and rest.

Leg cramps

Regular exercise can help you avoid leg cramps, too. You may find that sometimes you wake up in the night clutching your leg which is cramping painfully and have to walk around the room and massage it back to normal. Poor diet may be one cause although it is felt by some nutritionists that this cramping may sometimes be linked to drinking too much milk and a subsequent imbalance of calcium and magnesium in the body. However, it has also been suggested that too little calcium may also lead to cramp so you could try drinking a small glass of milk before you go to bed, perhaps with a magnesium or vitamin B6 supplement. Another way to ensure that you are getting adequate magnesium is to eat more leafy green vegetables.

If you do not eat enough salt, you may also suffer from cramp, especially in hot weather when you are inclined to sweat more. You do not need to eat large amounts of salt – let your appetite be your guide and just salt your food to taste, as too much salt can be equally bad for you.

If you feel that you cannot win on the diet front with so many conflicting theories, you can get comfort from the fact that exercise will stimulate circulation as discussed above, and this does prevent or limit cramping. Ankle and foot rotations improve blood flow in the area and the leg exercises shown here will be useful, too.

A final word about cramp: if you tend to get it at night, ensure that you keep your feet warm and covered, and do not pile too many heavy blankets on the bed – a duvet (continental quilt) is lighter and less trouble.

Pain in the legs

You may feel a variety of aches and pains in your legs during pregnancy ranging from just tired, aching muscles or muscle cramps to shooting, sharp pains and even sciatica. Gentle massage and resting and elevating the legs are the best remedies for general tiredness and soothing away aches and pains. However, towards the end of your pregnancy as the baby grows larger and heavier and your 'bump' shifts downwards in preparation for birth, you may experience sharp shooting pains, especially when you are walking. You may even have to stop and rest until the pain subsides. These pains may be caused by the increased pressure from the baby, especially after she engages. Slow breathing until the pain goes away followed by rest will help prevent these pains recurring. They may be a subtle warning that you are attempting too much and it is time to slow down and relax a little more. Make time each day to put your feet up at regular intervals.

Some pregnant women are amazed to feel sciatic pains in these last weeks. The pain is experienced in the sciatic nerve which continues from the lower back region through your bottom and down the outside of your legs. The most probable explanation for this is linked to the increased hormonal activity of progesterone in your body and the changes taking place in the softening of the ligaments in the spinal area. Rest, again, is the best remedy, especially supporting your thighs with cushions. Buttocks squeezing exercises may also be helpful. Practise these every day to relieve the pain.

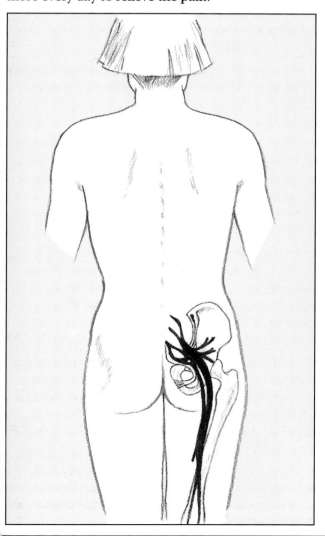

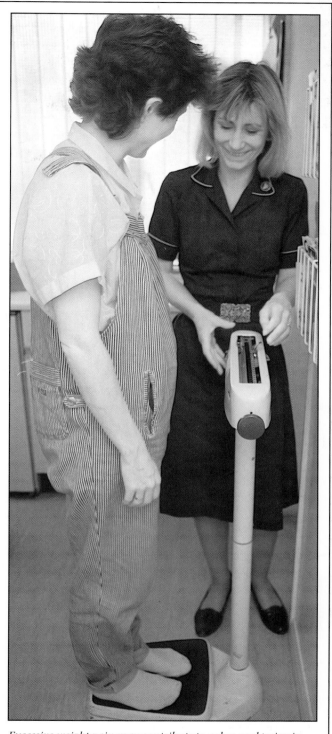

Excessive weight gain may contribute to aches and pains in your legs. Keeping within the boundaries of what constitutes acceptable weight gain will help relieve additional pressure on your legs. During the last weeks of pregnancy some women suffer from sciatic pain, and the position of the sciatic nerve is shown in the illustration on the left.

Run up a flattering loose pinafore

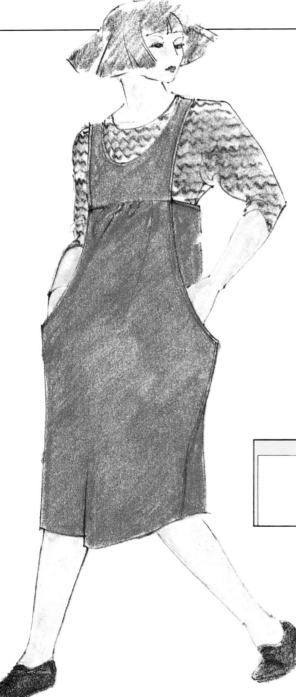

Materials
2.40m of 115cm fabric.

Size
To fit 14-16 (for size 12 trim 1.25cm off all side seams) 1sq = 5cm.

Cutting
Fold fabric in half lengthwise. Lay out pattern pieces using diagram as a guide. Cut two front top bodices to use one as a facing. 1.5cm seam allowances included in pattern.

To sew
With right sides together attach pocket facing to front body pocket openings. Trim and clip curve seam allowance, fold pocket facing to wrong side and topstitch 0.75cm from finished edge.

Gather upper edge front body to fit top, being careful not to catch in pocket facings.

Position front body over side panel with right sides both facing up matching pocket and markings. Baste around pocket and facing bag; stitch and neaten raw edge, leaving side seams open. Baste top of pocket and side seams to keep in place.

Place front top bodice pieces right sides together. Stitch around side and neck edges, leaving shoulder and lower edges open. Trim seams, clip curves. Turn to right side.

Join front body to top, right sides together between markings. Do not catch in top bodice facing.

Fold down seam allowance 1.5cm to wrong side on top of side panels. Turn in raw edge and topstitch across.

Press gathered seam allowance towards top bodice. Catch stitch top facing down over seam allowance on wrong side.

With right sides together, baste front to back between seam allowances at shoulder seams.

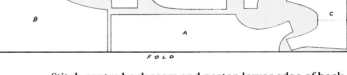

Stitch centre back seam and neaten lower edge of back facing.

With right sides together, pin back facing to back over front top.

Stitch armhole, shoulder and neck edges, being careful not to catch in front dress edges. Trim seams and corners; clip curves. Turn facing to inside; press.

With right sides together, stitch front to back at side seams, keeping back facing free; catch stitch down over side seam.

On right side, topstitch 0.75cm from neck and armhole edges. Turn up and stitch hem.

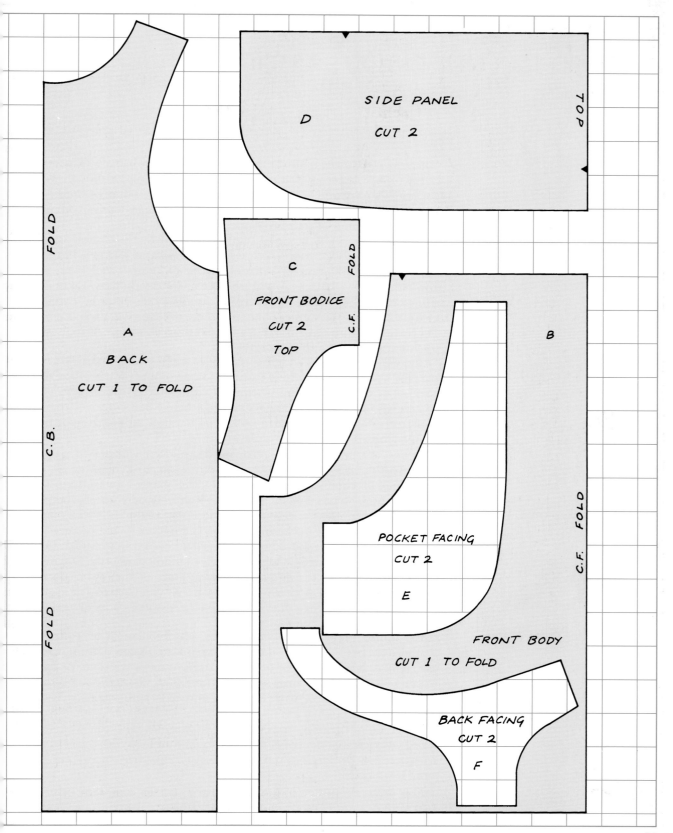

SIDE PANEL

D

CUT 2

TOP

FOLD

C.B.

FOLD

A

BACK

CUT 1 TO FOLD

C

FOLD

FRONT BODICE

CUT 2

TOP

C.F.

B

POCKET FACING

CUT 2

E

C.F. FOLD

FRONT BODY

CUT 1 TO FOLD

BACK FACING

CUT 2

F

Listen to your baby's heartbeat

You

You are well past the half-way mark now and are probably feeling on top of the world – bursting with health and well-being. Although you feel generally strong and active, do take notice of any bouts of tiredness and fatigue and put your feet up and rest a while. If these happen often have a word with your doctor just to be on the safe side.

Your 'bump' is still growing bigger and by now the top of your uterus will reach just above your navel. When your baby moves you may even be able to feel her different limbs through your abdominal wall. If you lie back and relax in the bath you will observe the extraordinary sight of your stomach moving as she twists inside you and delivers a few well-aimed kicks. When you next visit your clinic or doctor they will probably listen to her heartbeat through a fetal ear-trumpet or stethoscope. Have a listen-in, too, and hear her for the first time.

She will continue moving energetically when you sit down and relax or practise your deep-breathing exercises in readiness for the birth. You may also notice that she responds to music. You could try putting on a tape or record when you are reading or cooking – babies are supposed to respond well to classical music! It is very soothing to them, although some become extra vigorous when music is played.

In bed at night you may wake up more often – either to pass water because the baby may be pressing down on your bladder, or due to cramping in your legs and feet. This is a painful awakening and the affected limb needs instant massage from you or your partner. Heavy bedclothes can make it worse, so try sleeping under a duvet/continental quilt if you experience this annoying problem often. What you eat can also affect cramp, so you should try to make sure you drink enough fluid and have adequate salt, especially in the hot summer months. Doctors now know that too little salt and a low-sodium diet can be potentially dangerous to a baby. This does not mean that you have to salt everything heavily – far from it. Just salt your food to taste and let your appetite set its own limits.

Cramping may also be caused by an imbalance of calcium and magnesium in the body. You could try drinking a glass of milk before you go to bed with a supplement of magnesium or vitamin B6. Regular exercise will also help prevent it by stimulating circulation. Do some leg stretching rotation exercises every day and make sure you also have a daily brisk walk.

If you do get cramp, massage the calf muscles until the pain subsides. Keep your knee perfectly straight and hold your foot with the toes pointed *towards* you. For cramp in the foot, bend it upwards and massage firmly until it subsides.

You will also notice a drastic improvement in your skin. It will look better than ever as the pregnancy hormones continue their good work.

Keep it looking beautiful with regular cleansing, toning and moisturizing. If it looks good now you can ensure that it stays that way beyond the birth with adequate care and attention.

Your baby

She is growing fast now and measures about 33cm/13in long at the end of this month. Although her vital organs are quite mature she would look very thin indeed if she were born now. She has still to lay down fat deposits and plump out in readiness for birth. Her skin is becoming opaque and is no longer transparent and paper-thin. It still looks extremely wrinkled and is encased in its protective vernix covering.

Inside the womb the baby is getting used to all kinds of noises from the outside world as well as the sounds of your stomach rumbling and your heart beating. She can hear music, traffic noise, voices, the radio and TV and sometimes she sleeps through it all. This is all part of getting accustomed to sound and noise and probably accounts for how newborn babies can sleep peacefully through the loudest thunderstorm or in a nursery full of other crying, squealing infants.

Her ears started functioning two months ago and the amniotic fluid in which she is suspended carries sound well as there are no air cushions as yet to muffle any sound outside her eardrums. The amniotic fluid itself is renewed constantly and acts as a shock absorber for the baby's protection. Thus if you bump into something or fall down you are unlikely to harm the baby and should not worry. She is well cushioned against any knocks and bumps.

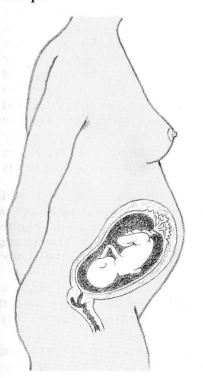

Rest . . . rest . . .
Now that you have entered the third and final trimester of your pregnancy you really must make time each day for rest and relaxation. This has spin-off benefits for labour in that it teaches you good breathing and how to relax and conserve energy. It also helps you avoid the late pregnancy-related problems of high blood pressure and toxaemia. And, of course, putting your feet up every day will ward off varicose veins and swelling in the feet and ankles. Even if you are still working, make sure that you rest regularly throughout the day, if only for 10-15 minutes at a time. When to rest? Try some deep-breathing exercises before you get up in the morning. Snatch some rest mid-morning with your fruit juice or coffee. Have a nap or deep relaxation session in the afternoon, and put your feet up after dinner.

Improve on nature with a new make-up

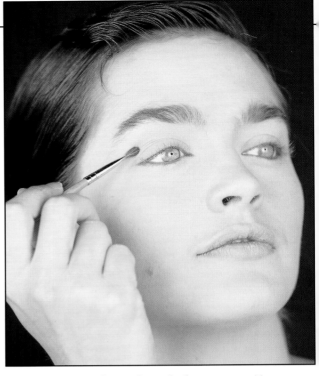

Eye make-up can be easily applied in minutes. Try experimenting with different techniques for a fresh, day-time face or a more elegant and sophisticated look.

Just because you are pregnant does not mean that you have to stop bothering about the way you look. Many women radiate such natural beauty during pregnancy that they explore the possibilities of a new make-up to enhance their improved skin and to make them feel good, too. For looking good is feeling good and will boost your confidence and improve your own body image.

The most important thing is to find a look with which you feel comfortable. Perhaps you have used the same old make-up for the last few years and now it looks rather dated or does not complement the new styles and fashions. It can be fun to experiment with new products and looks and you will be amazed at the results. Nowadays, make-up is not so much a matter of camouflaging one's faults but of creating a uniquely personal look, an individual style that is totally *you*.

When you are pregnant and feeling a little weary sometimes or slightly nauseous perhaps, you may not feel like spending a lot of time making-up your face. What you need is a quick, simple routine that is foolproof and always looks good. Keep to the same basics and you can vary the colours according to your mood or the occasion. And as we shall see, it is easy to transform your daytime face into a glamorous party look for evenings.

Invest in quality equipment

Your make-up will depend to some extent on the tools and equipment you use – the lighting, the mirror, the brushes, sponges and tissues. These need not be expensive and are a good investment for the future. For the best results, they are essential. You need the following basic items:

1   Good light – either natural or artificial. Never apply your make-up in the gloom where all colour looks subdued – the effect may be startling when you venture out into daylight. Try not to use fluorescent light either as this distorts true colours. Always make-up in plenty of natural light or by good incandescent lighting.

2   Use a hand mirror or a special make-up one on a stand. A magnifying mirror is useful for concealing shadows and making-up eyes.
3   You will need a large brush for applying loose powder; 3 or 4 small eye shadow brushes; a brush for putting on blusher and another for highlighting; a fine-line lip brush; a sponge for smoothing on foundation and some tissues and cotton wool. Do take good care of your brushes and sponges and wash them out frequently, preferably after use.

The rapid make-up routine

Use this basic routine in the morning when you are in a hurry. With practice, it should take no longer than 10 minutes to achieve your perfect look. Don't attempt to rush things initially. Wait until you have mastered the routine and you will find that you will soon speed up automatically.

1   Make-up begins with moisturizing
It is essential to apply make-up to a really well-cleansed skin which is thoroughly moisturized. This is most important in pregnancy when your skin has a natural tendency to be dry. The moisturizer will help

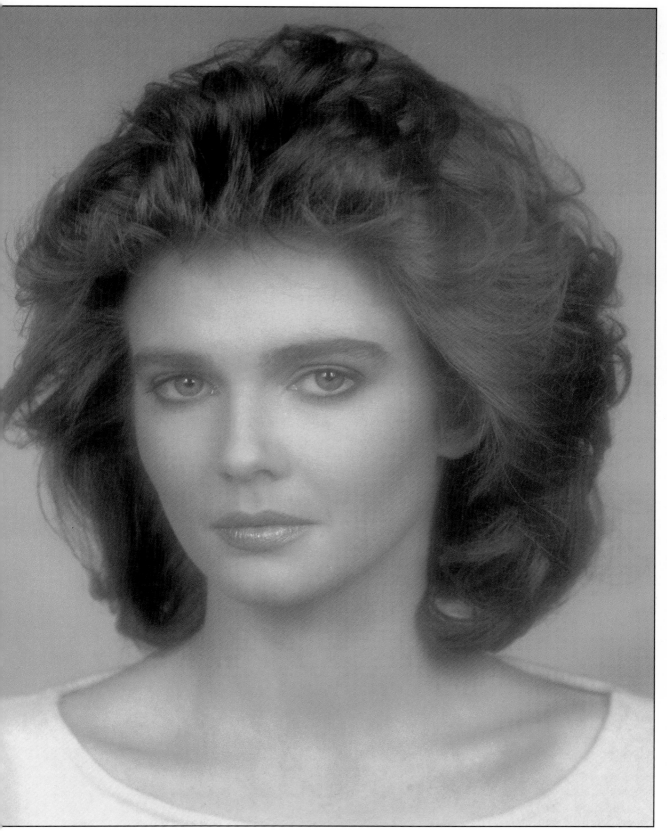

Improve on nature with a new make-up

protect your skin's natural moisture supplies and act as a barrier against the drying effects of sun, wind, cold, central heating and air conditioning. Use a light moisturizer that is quickly absorbed into the skin without it feeling slightly greasy.

In summer, you may prefer to use a tinted moisturizer instead of applying foundation on top. This gives a natural look and is ideal for showing off healthy, glowing skin which is unblemished. These products are particularly good for sport and exercise as they do not go cakey or streak. Some contain sunscreens for hot summer days. Choose one that is only one or two shades darker than your natural skin colour so that the result looks natural. Blend it in well round the jaw line.

2   Cover-up jobs
You may have some blemishes such as spots, broken veins, florid-looking skin or dark circles under the eyes that need concealing. You can buy special concealer sticks and creams for this purpose. They can be applied before or after smoothing in foundation. Pat gently into the skin and blend well. If you are using on the delicate skin under the eyes, be especially careful so as not to drag or damage it. It should blend into your natural skin tone. For a high

colour that needs toning down, you can use a green-tinted moisturizer. This will neutralize the skin tone and will be concealed by your foundation.

3   The foundations
Foundation is used to even out and improve the colour and texture of your skin. A good product can always improve on nature and make up for any deficiencies. Take time choosing the best foundation for your skin colour and type. Try a little out on your wrist first before buying as the colour on your skin rarely matches the one you see in the jar, which is more concentrated. If you are naturally pale, don't go for a deep bronze shade as it will look really bizarre. Here is a basic guide to help you choose:
Pale skins: choose a pinky or warm peach shade.
Medium skins: choose a rosy or peachy beige.
Dark skins: choose an olive or dark beige shade.
Of course, you can mix different shades together to get the perfect colour for you.

You can apply your foundation with the fingertips or a sponge. The latter gives a better, smoother finished look. It is important to blend it evenly all over the face and into the neck to avoid a colour line. Use sparingly, not thickly. You are aiming for a natural look – not a thick mask. The best way to apply it is to dot it across your face and then blend gently with a damp sponge.

4   Powder – the final dusting
A dusting of powder will 'set' your make-up and prolong it, helping you to stay looking fresher throughout the day. It will reduce shine and can be used when necessary to touch-up your foundation.

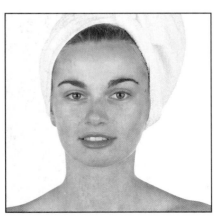

1 Cleanse your skin thoroughly and remove all your make-up. Tie your hair back off your face and study your skin and features.

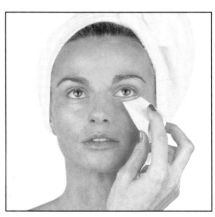

2 Using a damp make-up sponge, apply a light and even covering of foundation and gently blend into your neck and under the jaw.

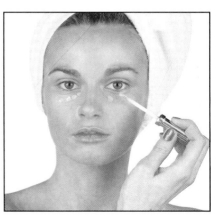

3 Dot the dark shadows under your eyes with a concealer liquid or stick and blend into your skin. Cover up any spots or blemishes.

Apply generously and then fluff away any excess with some cotton wool. Powders can be transparent, translucent, coloured, loose or compressed. A loose powder tends to look lighter than the compressed sort which is blended with foundation. Translucent powders are very flattering as they are light, have some colour but let the natural tone of your skin shine through. Of course, transparent ones do not add any colour at all.

5 Spotlight on your eyes

Many women consider their eyes to be their best feature and the focal point of their faces. Make-up can enhance the eyes' natural beauty and emphasize their colour and shape. It can be used to make narrow eyes look wider; big eyes less prominent; deep-set eyes more open; and closely-set eyes wider.

In later pregnancy your eyes may look a little puffy if you have a tendency to suffer from fluid retention. To alleviate this, you can try soaking two pads of cotton wool in witch hazel, squeezing them out and then lying down and relaxing for 10 minutes with a pad over each eye. Slices of cool cucumber placed over the eyes are also very effective.

Because you are eating a really healthy diet and drinking less (or no) alcohol, you will probably find that your eyes look clearer and less bloodshot. They look bright when you wake up in the mornings and don't feel heavy lidded. This is one of the great beauty spin-offs of being pregnant.

Make the most of your eyes with effective make-up. Always apply shadow and eyeliner first and then mascara to thicken and darken the lashes. Here's how to do it:

1 Apply eye shadow to the lid. Fairly neutral shades are usually best for daytime, such as browns, beiges, greys and greens, while more exciting shades of blue, gold, bronze, pink and violet are great for evening wear. Gently smooth a light shade into the lid and fade it out towards the eyebrows with a darker shade in the socket to define the shape of the eye. You can blend them together if wished for a smudged look. You can choose from powders, creams and glosses. As a general rule, creams look best, tend to last longer and do not crease into little crêpey lines like some powders. To emphasize the eyes, you can smudge a darker shade around the outer corners of the eye.

2 Outline and define the eyes with eyeliner or soft kohl pencil or crayon. You can choose from a wide range of colours including black, various shades of brown, grey, green and blue. Bright electric colours look good for parties and evenings out while more muted ones are better for day wear. Pencils look more natural than harsher lines and can be blended softly into the shadow on the upper lid and smudged at the corners. A hard, solid line of black eyeliner can be very ageing so it is better to opt for softer shades. For a mysterious look, you can follow the traditional method of many Eastern women and use a dark kohl pencil on the *inside* of the lower lids.

3 Mascara lends the finishing touches and makes the total effect look more glamorous. You may find that if your lashes tend to look clogged and heavy, it would be better to use a non-fibre mascara which builds up the lashes without any sticking together.

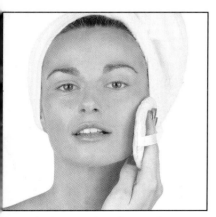

4 Apply the powder of your choice to 'set' your make-up and to help you look fresher. It will also reduce shine in the nose, forehead and chin areas.

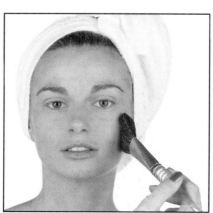

5 Gently apply some blusher along your cheekbones upwards towards your hairline. Aim for a subtle, natural hint of colour.

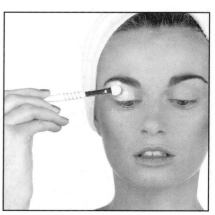

6 Apply eye shadow, powder or cream, to your lid. Neutral, subtle shades are better for daytime and brighter, more vivid colours for the evening.

Improve on nature with a new make-up

This type is also best on women with sensitive eyes. Stroke the lashes upwards and outwards on the upper lids to colour and curl them; and downwards and outwards on the lower lids. Remove any smudges from the surrounding skin with a tissue or some damp cotton wool. If you are going swimming or exercising, it may be a good idea to use a waterproof mascara which will not smudge or run. However, it is more difficult to remove and you should always use a specially formulated remover which will not stretch the tissues around the eyes.

6 Shape your lips

Lips need colour and definition but they should always balance your eyes. Don't over-stress one at the expense of the other. If you find that your lips tend to be dryer than usual during pregnancy you should use a rich moisturizing lipstick. You can define your lips' natural shape or change it with a lip pencil. Draw in the shape you desire with a brown-toned or pink lip pencil – you can use a brush if preferred for a finer result. Then fill in your lips with the colour of your choice. Soft, muted colours – beiges, corals, salmons and light pinks – are best for daytime. After applying a coat, blot well with tissue paper and then reapply. If your lipstick tends to 'bleed' around your mouth, you can powder it lightly after blotting.

For summer, translucent, pearly and glossy lipsticks look good in shimmering pinks. Lip glosses make evening lips shine, but creams are usually best for day wear. For a dramatic evening effect, you can experiment with deeper shades of red, fuchsia and plum or even shining golds and silvers, coppers and bronzes. You may wish to wear a shade that matches your outfit. It all depends on your natural colouring, your clothes and the occasion.

7 Shape and contour your face

Blusher, face shapers and highlighters can all redefine your face and add colour and interest. They have to be skilfully applied or the result may look unnatural and clumsy. Generally, a little blusher will accentuate daytime cheekbones, while shapers and highlighters are best kept for evenings when you wish to create a special effect.

If you have a tendency to be paler than usual in early pregnancy or the very last weeks before the birth, blusher can work wonders and give you a flattering touch of colour. Study your face in the mirror and smile to see the outlines of your cheekbones. Apply the blusher upwards along the bones towards the hairline. Be light with your touch and blend it softly into the surrounding skin. It should never stand out in unnatural spots of bright colour against a pale skin.

Blushers may be powders, creams or gels and the sort you use is mostly a matter of personal choice. Powder is OK for all skin types and easiest to apply, while creams tend to be most suitable for dry skins.

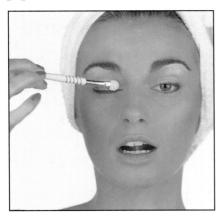

7 Gently smooth a light shade into the lid and fade it out towards the eyebrow. Use a darker shade in the socket to give more definition to the shape of the eye.

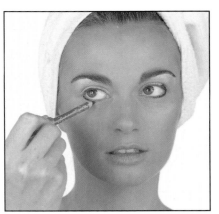

8 Outline the eyes with eyeliner or a soft kohl pencil. Blend this into the eye-shadow to avoid a hard, solid line of dark eyeliner. Mascara your lashes.

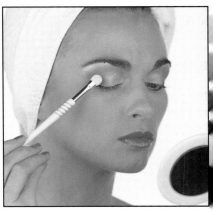

9 Outline your lips and fill them in with lipstick. Pat lightly and apply a second coat. Add the final finishing touches to achieve your finished look.

Gels give very sheer colour and are best kept for evenings or hot summer days worn over a tinted moisturizer. If you do not know which colour to choose, bear in mind that a basic peach suits most skin tones. Bright pinks, oranges and corals may look good on sallow or olive skins but *never* on pale complexions. You can use a brighter colour for evening, of course. One way to find the right shade is to pinch your cheeks gently to bring a spot of colour to your face. As this is your natural blush, it may be a good shade to aim for if you want a natural effect.

You can make light and shade work on your face with highlighters and contourers. These are often used to correct or minimize what you may perceive as faults. For example:

1   Apply a little shader to a double chin and fade it by blending well into the chin and neck area.

2   Make your nose look smaller by stroking some shader down the centre of your nose and blending lightly into the foundation at the sides.

3   Make your chin appear less pointed by dabbing a little shader onto the chin and blending it carefully into the neck.

Ivory highlighters are great for evening to make your face look really glamorous. A word of warning, however, they must be applied wisely or they will look very odd indeed! You can use them to widen eyes, to exaggerate cheekbones and add brightness and interest to eyes.

1   To make eyes appear wider, apply highlighter under brows.

2   To add brightness to eyes, dab a little highlighter onto the centre of your eyelids.

3   To exaggerate cheekbones, brush some highlighter across them.

Evening glamour

Natural-looking make-up which enhances your natural beauty in an understated way generally looks best for day wear, especially when you are pregnant and want to show off your radiant skin and looks. However, when the evening comes you can still change into a glamorous woman even with a 'bump'! You would be surprised at how many pregnant women look really attractive, especially when they are looking dazzling at a party in sensational evening make-up and a beautiful flowing dress.

You do not have to strip off your daytime make-up and start again with fresh, although you can if you

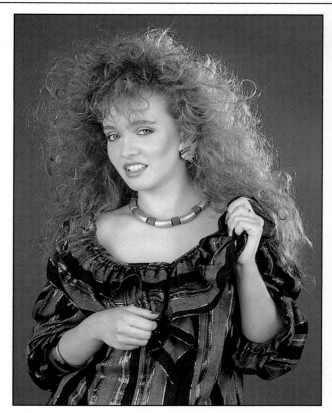

You can easily create a glamorous evening face by using brighter, more vivid eye colours and lipstick, and adding gloss and shine.

wish, of course. Sometimes it is refreshing to cleanse your face thoroughly and reapply make-up before going out in the evening. If you don't have time for this, you can still transform your face into a glamorous party look by adding colour to your daytime make-up. A brighter blusher, highlighters and glosses will make your skin glow, whereas iridescent eye shadows in gold, silver, pink or deep, bright colours will emphasize your eyes. Touch up your eyeliner and apply another coat of mascara on top of the old. A dusting of translucent, shimmery powder will 'set' your face. Smooth in a brighter, glossier shade of lipstick and you will be ready for the sun. All this need take only five minutes.

For the finishing touches and to boost your confidence, spray or dab on a little of your favourite scent. You can use a lighter *eau-de-toilette* or *eau-de-parfum* during the day and a headier *parfum* in the evening. Floral fragrances are soft, romantic and lighter for daytime wear; green, woody, perfumes are sporty and business-like; oriental, spicy scents are particularly sensual and glamorous.

Getting the right nutrients in your diet

Stock up on nutrients

You are now aware how important it is to eat a varied diet which supplies all the nutrients you and your baby need for good health. But do you know the best sources and how to cook delicious meals that are high in, say, iron or protein? And did you realize that some nutrients are better absorbed and used by the body when eaten in combination with others – for example, more iron is absorbed when eaten in conjunction with vitamin C. Eating these dishes regularly will give you the confidence that you are getting the nutrients you need. Of course, they are only suggestions and you can probably think of hundreds of ways of supplying your daily intake of nutritional goodness. The recipes below have been chosen with the following criteria in mind – supplying a well-balanced dish, which can be prepared and cooked easily and quickly with the minimum of fuss. Neither are they expensive.

Calcium

You need calcium for your baby's developing skeleton and teeth, and to strengthen your own, too. If you do not get enough of this mineral your baby may draw on your supply and you may find that you end up in the dentist's chair as a result. During the last three months of your pregnancy your need for calcium will be greater than ever. If you are deficient, you may experience leg cramps, headaches and find it difficult to sleep. Adequate calcium will also help form your child's future good looks by building strong facial bones and teeth. When it is insufficient, teeth may be crooked or crowded and jaws poorly formed.

Like iron, only a small amount of the calcium you eat passes into your bloodstream for use by the body. If your diet is poor, your stomach may not produce enough hydrochloric acid to dissolve the calcium for absorption. And although it is tempting to drink skimmed rather than whole milk during pregnancy to avoid putting on unwanted weight, the calcium in whole milk is better absorbed due to its cream and lactose content.

You do not have to just drink plenty of milk to ensure an adequate supply of calcium. Cheese, buttermilk, sardines, eggs, beans, yoghurt and leafy green vegetables also supply this mineral.

Sardine salad

2 cans sardines in oil
1 cucumber, sliced and salted, rinsed and drained
1 onion, sliced thinly in rings
60ml/4 tablespoons French dressing
15ml/1 tablespoon lemon juice
225g/8oz cooked long-grain brown rice
5ml/1 teaspoon turmeric
1 bunch watercress
30ml/2 tablespoons chopped parsley

Drain the sardines and set aside. Put the cucumber and onion in a dish with the French dressing and lemon juice. Colour the rice yellow by gently forking in the turmeric and place in a serving dish with the onion and cucumber on top. Arrange the sardines in a star shape fanning out from the centre. Make a border of watercress sprigs and sprinkle with parsley. Serves 4.

Broccoli mornay

450g/1lb broccoli spears
4 slices ham
25g/1oz/⅛ cup butter
25g/1oz/¼ cup flour
300ml/½ pint/1¼ cups milk
good pinch ground nutmeg
squeeze lemon juice
2.5ml/½ teaspoon mustard
100g/4oz/⅔ cup grated hard cheese

Cook the broccoli in boiling salted water until just tender. Drain and arrange in a greased ovenproof dish with the slices of ham. Make a white sauce: melt the butter and stir in the flour. Cook gently over low heat for 2-3 minutes without browning. Gradually add the milk, beating until smooth. Bring to the boil, stirring constantly and then season. Add the nutmeg, lemon juice, mustard and half the cheese. Pour over the broccoli and sprinkle with the remaining cheese. Dot the top with butter and place under a hot grill until golden and bubbling *or* bake in a preheated oven at 200°C, 400°F, gas 6 until golden-brown. Makes 2-3 servings.

Iron

During pregnancy it is absolutely essential that you get an adequate supply of iron. You will probably be prescribed a course of iron tablets, and it is a good idea to eat liver once or twice a week as this is remarkably rich in iron. Liver and kidney are the best foods to eat, and even if you do not enjoy the taste, there are many ways to disguise the flavour and make them more interesting.

Much of the iron you take in is not used by the body, and eating a source of vitamin C at the same meal will help its absorption.

Italian chicken liver risotto

1 onion, chopped
1 clove garlic, crushed
4 rashers streaky bacon, chopped
45ml/3 tablespoons oil
225g/8oz/1 cup brown long-grain rice
550ml/1 pint/2½ cups chicken stock
1 small packet saffron
chopped fresh herbs (basil, oregano)
salt and pepper
100g/4oz mushrooms, sliced
225g/8oz chicken livers
seasoned flour
25g/1oz/⅛ cup butter
juice and grated rind of 1 orange
40g/1½oz/¼ cup grated Parmesan cheese
chopped parsley to garnish

Sauté the onion, garlic and bacon in the oil until soft and golden. Stir in the rice until every grain is glistening with oil. Pour in some of the stock and bring to the boil. Reduce to a bare simmer, add the saffron, herbs, seasoning and mushrooms. Cook gently until the rice is tender, adding more stock as and when necessary. Stir frequently to prevent the rice sticking. Towards the end, dust the chicken livers with flour and fry in the butter until golden. Slice and mix into the risotto with the orange rind and juice. Season to taste and serve with Parmesan and parsley. Makes 4 servings.

Calves' liver alla pizzaiola

60ml/4 tablespoons olive oil
1 onion, sliced
3 cloves garlic, crushed
450g/1lb tomatoes, skinned and chopped
5ml/1 teaspoon chopped oregano or basil
675g/1½lb calves' liver, very thinly sliced
chopped parsley to garnish

Heat half the olive oil in a pan and sauté the onion and garlic until soft. Add the tomatoes and herbs and bring to the boil. Cook over a medium heat until the sauce reduces and thickens. Season with salt and plenty of ground black pepper. Meanwhile, remove the skin from the liver and cut out any gristly bits. Heat the remaining oil and when it is very hot, add the liver. Cook very fast and turn it over as soon as it stops looking red and raw. Cook the other side quickly and serve in the tomato sauce sprinkled with plenty of fresh chopped parsley. The liver should still be slightly pink inside and tender. Overcooking will cause it to be tough. Serves 4.

Orange spinach salad

350g/12oz spinach, washed and trimmed
6 chicken livers, sliced
15ml/1 tablespoon oil
4 rashers streaky bacon, crisply grilled/broiled
60ml/4 tablespoons French dressing
2 oranges
chopped chives

Prepare the spinach and place in a bowl. Sauté the chicken livers in the oil until golden and mix with the spinach. Crumble the bacon over the top and mix well with the French dressing. Season. Remove all the peel and white pith from the oranges. Slice across horizontally and arrange on top of the salad. Sprinkle with chives. Makes 3-4 servings.

Protein

You will remember that protein comes not only from meat and animal products (cheese, milk, yoghurt, eggs, fish) but also from some vegetables and pulses. Beans are particularly high in protein, especially soya beans, and have the advantage of being very cheap and tasty and also a good source of B vitamins and dietary fibre. If you do not have the time to cook and soak dried beans, you can always open a can of baked beans for a nutritious snack. An average 225g/8oz can contains about 12 grams of protein. Served on wholemeal bread with an egg and ham or bacon, the count nearly doubles.

Here are some ideas you may not have thought of for including protein in your diet to complement the meat, fish, poultry, eggs and cheese.

Getting the right nutrients in your diet

Lasagne

300ml/½ pint/1¼ cups white sauce
8-12 sheets lasagne
50g/2oz/⅓ cup freshly grated Parmesan cheese
15g/½oz/1 tablespoon butter
Ragù sauce:
1 onion, chopped
1 clove garlic, crushed
1 carrot, diced
1 stick celery, diced
30ml/2 tablespoons oil
225g/8oz ground/minced beef
150ml/¼ pint/⅝ cup red wine (optional)
salt and pepper
100ml/4floz/½ cup milk
2.5ml/½ teaspoon ground nutmeg
450g/1lb tomatoes, skinned and chopped (or canned)
15ml/1 tablespoon sugar
good pinch of oregano

Make the ragù sauce: sauté the onion, garlic, carrot and celery in the oil until tender. Add the beef and cook quickly until faintly browned. Pour in the wine and seasoning and cook until the wine has evaporated.

Add the milk and nutmeg and continue cooking until absorbed. Add the tomatoes, sugar and oregano and turn up the heat until the tomatoes start bubbling and the sauce thickens a little. Reduce to a bare simmer and cook gently for about two hours, stirring occasionally, until reduced and richly coloured.

Make the white sauce. Then cook the lasagne sheets in boiling salted water until tender. Drain and pat dry. Assemble the lasagne in a buttered gratin dish. Put a little hot ragù in the bottom and cover with pasta, then another layer of meat sauce topped with some white sauce. Continue layering in this way until all the pasta and sauces are used up, ending with a layer of white sauce. Sprinkle with plenty of grated Parmesan and dot with butter.

Bake in a preheated oven at 230°C, 450°F, gas 8

for 20 minutes until the lasagne is bubbling and golden-brown. Serve hot with a green salad or French beans. This dish freezes successfully. Makes 4 servings.

Bean and pasta soup

1 onion, chopped
2 cloves garlic, crushed
4 large carrots, sliced
3 sticks celery, sliced
30ml/2 tablespoons oil
1 litre/1¾ pints/4½ cups stock
400g/14oz canned tomatoes
15ml/1 tablespoon tomato paste
salt and pepper
pinch sugar
chopped basil or oregano
225g/8oz cooked red kidney beans
100g/4oz spaghetti or noodles
grated Parmesan cheese to serve

Sauté the onion, garlic, carrot and celery in the oil until tender and golden. Add the stock, tomatoes, tomato paste, seasoning, sugar and herbs. Bring to the boil and then reduce the heat to a simmer. Cook gently for about 1 hour with the pan covered. Add the beans and pasta and cook gently for 15-20 minutes, or until the pasta is tender. Serve in soup bowls sprinkled with freshly grated Parmesan cheese. Makes 6 servings.

Vitamin C
If you eat plenty of fresh fruit and vegetables and drink fruit juices in preference to soft drinks, then you probably get enough vitamin C. However, it is still a good idea to include some dishes that are valuable sources in your diet and to consume some at every meal to ensure that you maintain a constant level in your bloodstream all day long. Eating all your vitamin C at breakfast-time or just taking a pill daily will not ensure an adequate supply.

In order to do this you could have a glass of orange juice or half a grapefruit for breakfast; some salad for lunch; a green vegetable for dinner; and fresh fruit to munch between meals. It is really very simple. As vitamin C is destroyed easily (by smoking, alcohol and aspirin, for instance) you must take special care. Avoid those substances that may interfere with your body's supply, and take special care when preparing food and vegetables. As soon as they are cut open

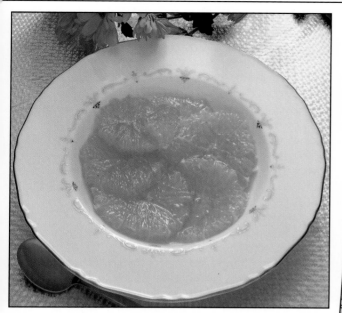

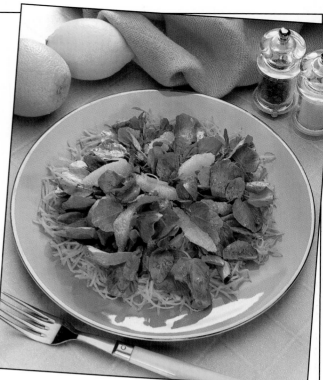

Caramel oranges and Watercress and orange salad are appetitising ways to increase your daily vitamin C intake and make a pleasant change from eating the fruit alone.

and exposed to the air their vitamin C content starts to diminish. Boiling or adding baking soda to the cooking water can destroy the vitamin C in vegetables. Always steam them for preference or cook very quickly by popping them into already boiling water and eating while firm and crisp.

Eating a piece of fresh fruit is one of the simplest ways to finish off a meal. Ring the changes with these desserts, all rich in vitamin C.

Summer fruit salad

2 large oranges, peeled and segmented
1 ruby red grapefruit, peeled and segmented
225g/8oz strawberries, hulled and sliced
100g/4oz raspberries
100g/4oz redcurrants, trimmed
100ml/4floz/½ cup fresh orange juice

Prepare the fruit and place in a bowl. Cover with orange juice and serve with natural yoghurt and flaked toasted almonds if wished. Serves 3-4.

Watercress and orange salad

4 oranges
finely grated carrot (optional)
3 large bunches watercress, washed and trimmed

7½ tablespoons vegetable oil
juice and rind of 1 orange
pinch sugar
1¼ teaspoons lemon juice
salt and pepper

Remove the peel and pith from the oranges. Segment the orange, reserving any juice. Lay the grated carrot on a plate and arrange the orange and watercress on top. Add the remaining ingredients to the orange juice and pour over the salad. Serves 4.

Caramel oranges

4 large juicy oranges
juice of 2 oranges
25g/1oz/⅛ cup soft brown sugar

Remove all the peel and pith from the oranges and cut across horizontally into thin slices. Arrange in a dish. Squeeze out any remaining juice from the outer peel pieces into a pan together with the juice of two fresh oranges. If wished, cut a little peel into very thin strips and place in the pan also. Add the sugar and stir over very low heat to dissolve completely. Boil for a minute or two and then pour over the oranges. Cool and serve chilled. Makes 2 servings.

Shape up with your antenatal work-out

You will know by now that pregnancy is not the right time to try out new forms of exercise. Any exercises should be gentle, controlled, simple movements. They should be carried out slowly and methodically, and should gradually stretch and strengthen muscles and joints. As well as promoting fitness, the exercises emphasise awareness and control. Integration of body and mind prepares a woman for labour when her body is doing all the work but she has to be in control of the situation mentally and emotionally.

By this stage of your pregnancy exercise programme, your figure will be changing shape and you should be aware of how changes affect your physical capabilities. Listen to any messages that your body gives you to slow down. Do not push it beyond its natural limits – you are the best judge of

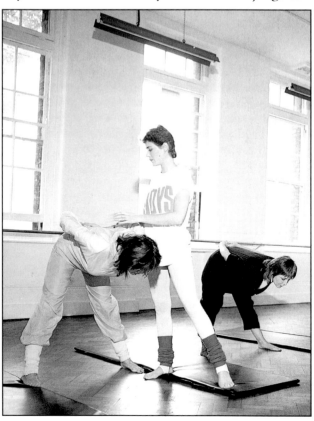

what is right for you. You will probably find that exercise during pregnancy will actually heighten your body awareness.

Aim for quality – not quantity. Do not over-work nor over-stretch muscles and do not expect your body to work and respond as it did in its pre-pregnancy state. You are twice as likely as usual to fall prey to backache so avoid any exercises that will strain your back. Check your posture when you exercise, as your spinal ligaments soften during pregnancy and the increased weight of your abdomen with the placenta and growing baby put additional strain on your back.

Correct technique is very important when performing pregnancy exercises so that you do not strain or damage any muscles or put extra stress on your body. Always follow the instructions carefully and do not be tempted to go beyond them – to perform more repetitions than is recommended, to stretch further than is advised or to introduce new exercises that are not specifically part of an antenatal programme. And remember to breathe naturally and easily when exercising. Do not hold your breath or over-breathe.

Your hormonal balance will affect your exercise performance during pregnancy, too. Increased progesterone and oestrogen help to relax muscles and contribute to fluid retention and poor circulation. Rhythmic movements, on the other hand, improve circulation, strengthen muscles and make joints more flexible, especially if extra fluid in the body makes them stiff. So you can see that regular, controlled exercise has far-reaching benefits for your health, level of fitness, flexibility and your eventual delivery.

By now you should have a comprehensive exercise routine that you practise carefully and regularly. It should include a warm-up prior to the exercise programme proper, and then specific exercises for working the upper body (arms, chest), the waist and lower body (abdomen, legs and hips), followed by relaxation.

Most antenatal classes are a mixture of special pregnancy related exercises and relaxation as shown here. The exercises are gentle but should be

Dress comfortably when you work-out during pregnancy – a loose sweatshirt or T-shirt, and tights or soft trousers with an expanding maternity waistline or panel are ideal. Wear socks or legwarmers to keep feet and leg muscles warm while exercising. This helps reduce the risk of injuries.

Side leg raise

1 Lie on your right side and point the toes of your top leg downwards.
2 Concentrating on your hip and outer thigh muscles, slowly lift the left leg upwards, keeping the toes pointing downwards.

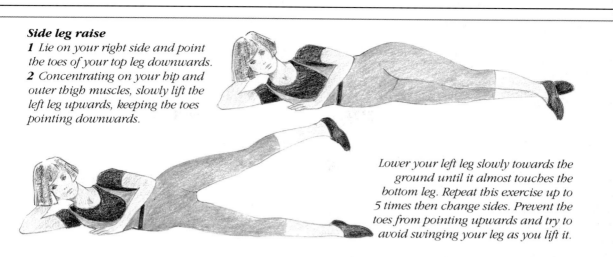

Lower your left leg slowly towards the ground until it almost touches the bottom leg. Repeat this exercise up to 5 times then change sides. Prevent the toes from pointing upwards and try to avoid swinging your leg as you lift it.

Kneeling squat

1 Start in a kneeling position, with your arms held out in front of you at shoulder level.
2 Slowly lower your buttocks towards the floor, keeping your body straight to avoid knee stress. Return to the starting position and continue this up and down movement. Do 10 repetitions.

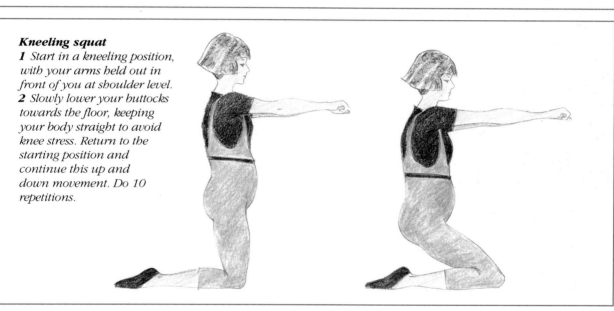

Side leg lift

1 Lie on your right side with your left knee bent and tucked behind your right leg, and your left foot flat on the floor. Lean on your right elbow and support your head with your hand.

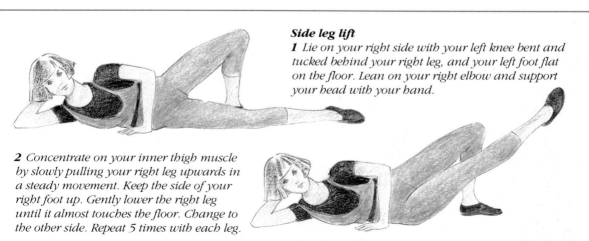

2 Concentrate on your inner thigh muscle by slowly pulling your right leg upwards in a steady movement. Keep the side of your right foot up. Gently lower the right leg until it almost touches the floor. Change to the other side. Repeat 5 times with each leg.

Shape up with your antenatal work-out

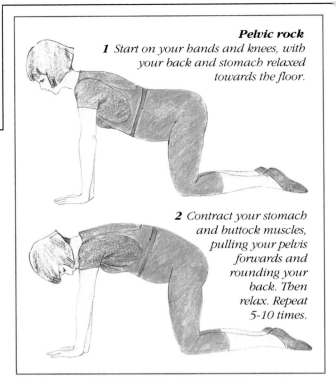

Pelvic rock

1 Start on your hands and knees, with your back and stomach relaxed towards the floor.

2 Contract your stomach and buttock muscles, pulling your pelvis forwards and rounding your back. Then relax. Repeat 5-10 times.

practised regularly for maximum effect. It is reassuring to exercise with other mothers-to-be, and there is an air of comradeship and friendly support. It is important to make yourself comfortable with mats and pillows or cushions while you go through the exercise routine. The instructor will check that you are performing the exercises correctly and is on hand to advise you and answer your questions concerning the safety of a particular exercise. Often she is a qualified midwife and will be able to talk over more general pregnancy problems, too. There may be a talk or class discussion on various aspects of pregnancy and labour as well as babycare when the exercise and relaxation session is over. This is a good opportunity for you to air any worries you may have and to share your experiences with others.

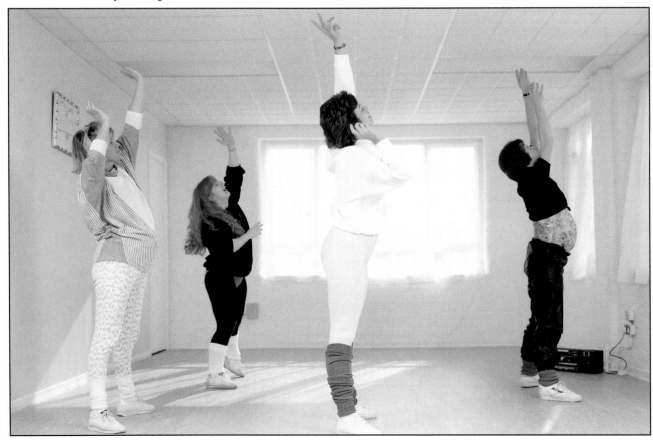

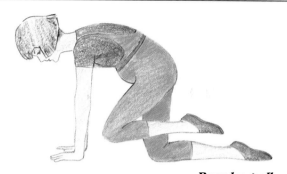

Rear leg pull

1 Start on your hands and knees, and slowly pull one leg up and inwards towards your stomach.

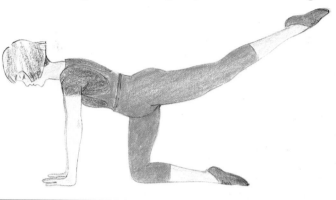

2 Extend your leg slowly, lifting it back and outwards. Return to the starting position and repeat. Feel the lower part of your buttocks tighten as the leg is extended. Repeat 3-4 times with each leg.

Knee lift

1 Start on your hands and knees with palms flat on floor in front of you, shoulder width apart.

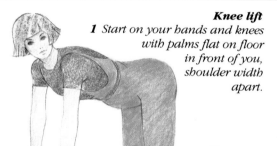

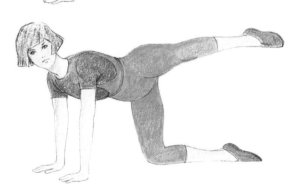

2 Lift one leg up to the side, using hip and outer thigh muscles and keeping the knee bent. Avoid swinging your leg out of control. Lower to start position and repeat. Change legs and start the exercise again.

Back arch

1 Lie on your back with your arms extended 90° out to the sides, palms downwards. Bend your knees and keep your feet flat on the floor.

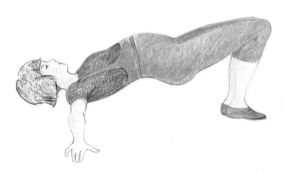

2 Slowly raise hips and your lower back upwards until the back is in a straight line. Avoid over-arching. Tighten your buttocks as you lift your hips. Repeat 3-6 times.

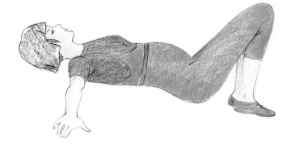

Run up a glamorous evening dress

This month we show you how to make a glamorous evening dress in which you can feel a million dollars. You can team it up with a sparkling sequinned jacket for really special occasions, some fashionable costume jewellery or some gold or silver evening shoes (preferably with not too high a heel). With the advantages of healthy, glowing skin and glossy hair, you can really sparkle at parties and dinners. If you prefer to buy an evening dress or outfit, you may find some garments in dramatic velvets, sumptuous silks and satins, or dazzling gold lurex. If they are cut to hang loosely, they may be equally suitable for ordinary wear as well as pregnancy wear. You need not spend a fortune either. There are lots of cut-price chic clothes that would meet these requirements in the large fashion chains and big department stores, and it is worth spending the time looking for them.

You do not have to shop exclusively in maternity stores. Many designers now have ranges that incorporate chic but suitably flowing or loose dresses, coats, jackets and tops. Shop around and you may be surprised at what you find.

Evening dress

Materials
3.5m of 115cm fabric. You will need extra if it has a one way design or nap. No-sewing press stud.

Size
To fit 12-16. Back length 116cm. 1.5cm seam allowance included in pattern. 1sq = 5cm.

Cutting
Make pattern pieces for back, right front and left front using squared diagram carefully following the appropriate marked lines. Open out fabric with right side facing you, cut right and left fronts using layout diagram as a guide. Fold remaining fabric and cut as diagram.

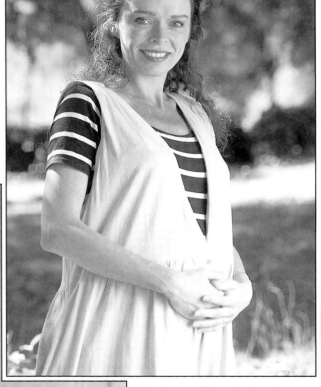

The dresses (left and above) are loose and casual enough to be worn every day but also suitable and sufficiently smart for work. As shown opposite, maternity dresses are now very fashionable and come in a wide range of styles, colours and fabrics to give you the widest possible choice.

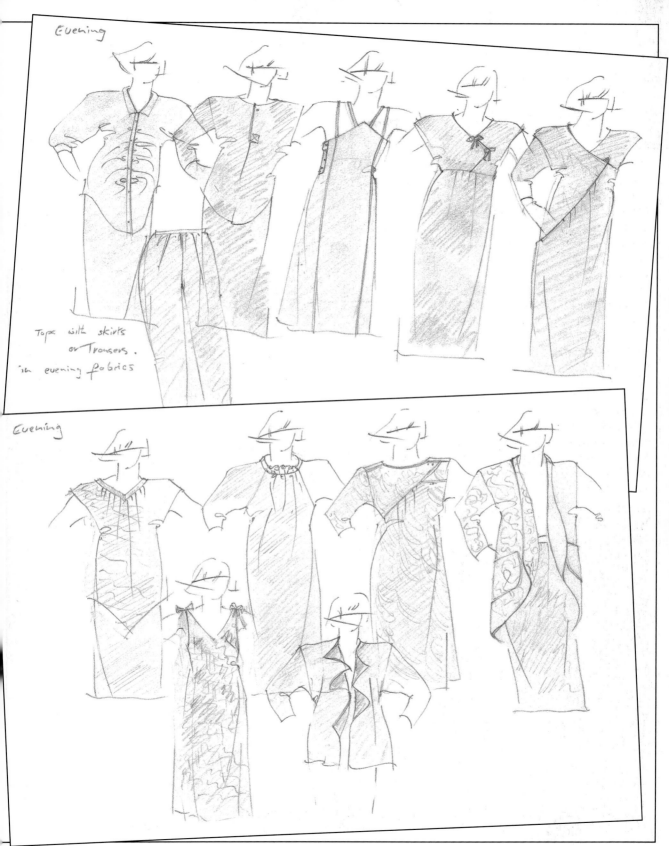

Evening

Tops with skirts
or Trousers.
in evening fabrics

Evening

Run up a glamorous evening dress

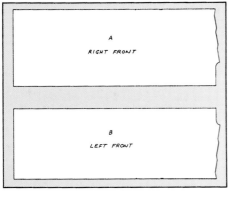

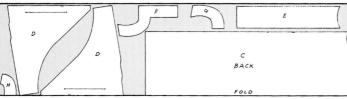

To sew

Join sleeve sections to back and fronts matching markers with right sides together, stitch to dot. Press seam towards body.

Pleat front and back sections as indicated on pattern, facing pleats away from front and back centres. Stitch shoulder panels to back with right sides together then stitch on fronts.

Stitch facings together at back shoulder seams. Fold right front back along fold line so that right sides of fabric are facing. Join on right front facing. Stitch facings to neck edge from right front. Fold round back, left front neck and down left front seam to dot.

Snip seam allowance on left front to dot as marked on pattern.

Turn facings over to wrong side and press.

Stitch left and right fronts together from dot. Fold right front on fold line over left front to form pleat 4cm wide matching centre front markers. Stitch across lower end of front opening and again 1.5cm above as marked on pattern. With right sides together join side and sleeve seams. Hem sleeves and dress. Fasten on studs as marked on pattern.

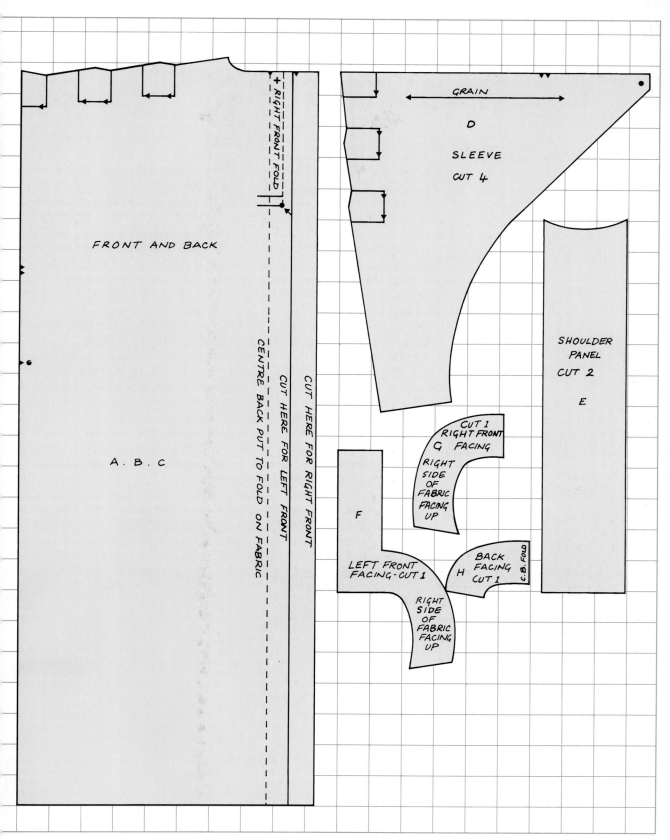

FRONT AND BACK

A . B . C

RIGHT FRONT FOLD

CUT HERE FOR LEFT FRONT

CENTRE BACK PUT TO FOLD ON FABRIC

CUT HERE FOR RIGHT FRONT

GRAIN

D

SLEEVE

CUT 4

SHOULDER
PANEL
CUT 2

E

CUT 1
RIGHT FRONT
G FACING

RIGHT
SIDE
OF
FABRIC
FACING
UP

F

LEFT FRONT
FACING - CUT 1

RIGHT
SIDE
OF
FABRIC
FACING
UP

BACK
FACING
CUT 1

H

C.B. FOLD

113

Play soothing music to your child

You

You are now entering the last trimester of your pregnancy at the end of which you will meet your baby. However, there is no reason why you should stop working now if you feel strong and well, nor should you abandon your regular exercise programme. From now on, you may slow down a little although not all women do. For example, you may feel a little breathless when you climb a couple of flights of stairs. Do not worry about this – if you start to puff, just slow down and take a few deep breaths. Breathing correctly and deeply is important now as the baby gets larger and you discover that you tend automatically to draw shallower breaths than usual.

At your antenatal classes, which you should be attending by now, especially if this is your first baby, you will be taught breathing exercises in readiness for labour, along with conscious relaxation techniques. Whether you are planning a 'natural' drug-free birth or otherwise, it will be a great help in labour if you can breathe and pant your way through the contractions. Although this will not eliminate any pain, it will make it more bearable and enable you to feel more in control of your body, less tense and more relaxed. Sometimes partners are encouraged to accompany you to these classes in order that they may gain an understanding of parenthood and even learn to 'coach' you through your labour, offering practical help and support.

Meanwhile, in your body great changes are continuing to take place and its familiar shape is fast disappearing as your abdomen swells. Your breasts are probably quite enlarged by now and may look veined and feel heavy. A little clear colostrum may even leak from the nipples. Continue washing and drying them daily and rub in a little lanolin or vitamin E based cream to

During your last three months of pregnancy you should take particular care to slow down and have regular rests each day. Give yourself plenty of time when doing any tasks, moving around, or travelling from one place to another. If you are in a full time job this is a good point to stop working, unless you still feel full of energy and health. You will probably feel your baby kicking fairly regularly and may even be able to distiguish her limbs as your stomach moves.

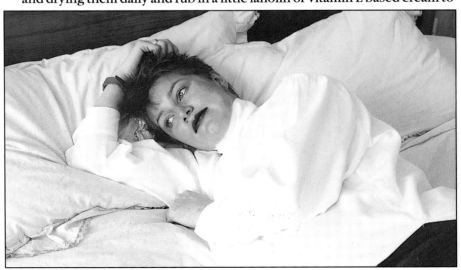

maintain their suppleness, prevent sore nipples and fight off stretch marks. You may have to invest in a new, larger bra to support their growing weight – a light cotton fabric is most comfortable. It can be used for breastfeeding later on, too, if it unfastens at the front.

You may begin to feel uncomfortable from the increased pressure on your stomach, intestine and diaphragm as your 'bump' gets bigger. This often causes heartburn, especially at night after dinner. Follow the guidelines for avoiding it – smaller meals, fewer spicy and fried foods, no late dinners and sitting upright, not slumping.

You may find that you are aware of your baby moving right through the day now, although many working and busy mothers hardly notice this until they sit down and put their feet up in the evenings. If your partner puts his hand on your abdomen, he may feel the baby kicking, too. In fact, when you lie back and relax in the bath, you may even be able to see the baby moving about as your abdomen rises and falls and sways from side to side. Some women can even distinguish a foot, an elbow or a bottom!

Your baby

If your baby was born now, she would stand a reasonable chance of survival despite her early arrival. Most babies born prematurely at seven months have at least a sixty per cent chance of life. Most of the available space in your uterus is now being taken up by the baby and soon she will turn into a head-down position in readiness for the birth. When this happens, she will fit a little more comfortably, although it will not be until she actually descends into the pelvis that you will really feel lighter.

By week 31, your baby will weigh about 1.8kg/4lb, and her appearance is less strange and more human as her head is more in proportion to her body. She is already laying down stores of fat and is filling out fast. Her weight will more or less double by the time she is born in less than three months' time. She is now covered all over with vernix, a greasy substance which affords her some protection against the surrounding amniotic fluid in which she is suspended.

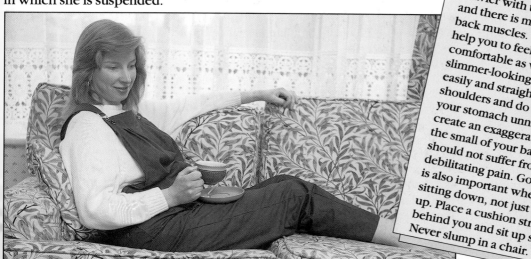

Watch your posture
If you have not encountered backache so far in your pregnancy, you are more likely to experience it now when your abdomen is getting larger and heavier with the growing baby and there is more strain on your back muscles. Good posture will help you to feel more comfortable as well as taller and slimmer-looking. If you walk easily and straight with relaxed shoulders and do not thrust out your stomach unnaturally to create an exaggerated hollow in the small of your back, you should not suffer from this debilitating pain. Good posture is also important when you are sitting down, not just standing up. Place a cushion strategically behind you and sit up straight. Never slump in a chair.

Treat your face and feet to a beauty session

'Oh, my aching feet!' is a familiar cry during pregnancy. It's not surprising that feet get sore and tired sometimes when you consider that they have to support the extra weight you are carrying around. They suffer particularly in the later months, perhaps after a long shopping expedition or a strenuous walk.

Feet are easily overlooked in your daily beauty routine and years of neglect can create many problems. If you usually slip your feet into ill-fitting shoes at the beginning of the day and then forget about them until tell-tale aches and pains appear, then it is time to reform and take better care of them. The golden rule to remember is: take care of your feet and they will be loyal to you.

Foot problems can contribute to a general feeling of fatigue and you can do without this during pregnancy. All your body weight is supported by just 26 small bones in each foot and powerful ligaments and muscles. Your feet are very tough as there are four muscle layers in the soles alone. However, neglect can lead to corns, hard skin, callouses, bunions and other irritations, and there is nothing like one of these to make you feel tired and low.

Beautifully healthy feet need regular exercise, comfortable, well-fitting shoes and beauty care if they are to stay that way. Pregnancy is a good time to start caring for them. If you rarely exercise, lead a sedentary lifestyle and tend to drive everywhere you may develop slack muscles and poor circulation in your feet and this can lead, in turn, to fallen arches, corns and callouses.

Wearing the right shoes

Your choice of footwear is very important during pregnancy. You should opt for low, comfortable shoes which will exercise your foot and leg muscles properly, help circulation and prevent the formation of ugly varicose veins. As your abdomen gets larger and your weight is inevitably directed forwards, you need flat shoes to keep your body supported and well-balanced. High heels tend to make you shift

your weight even further forwards and can cause backache as well as tired feet. Because they throw your posture off balance, the pelvis is tilted in such a way that the sacral muscles at the base of the spine go into spasm. An exaggerated hollowed back and lower back pain are indicative of poor posture and badly fitting high heeled shoes. You can do without these in pregnancy.

Comfortable shoes should fit properly with plenty of room for your toes. They should not rub your heels, be too tight, too narrow, too small nor too pointed. It may be difficult to buy exactly the right fitting for your feet as manufacturers have tended to standardize sizes and fittings and the general trend has been towards narrower shoes. You may have to shop around and try on several pairs before you find some shoes that feel really comfortable as well as looking good *and* flattering your feet. Do not be swayed by the talk of sales assistants and the bland assurances that the leather will stretch and that you can 'break them in'. Although leather will give and stretch a little, shoes should fit properly when you first try them on. If they don't, the likelihood is that they never will. If the shoes feel uncomfortable in any way, try another pair on instead.

Any pressure on your toes can lead to corns and bunions. And, as already shown, badly fitting shoes can cause backache, leg problems, fatigue and even cellulite build-up on thighs. The best time to buy shoes is during the afternoon when your feet tend to be more tired and swollen than first thing in the morning. If the shoes feel comfortable then, you know that they will stay that way.

Luckily, flat shoes are now fashionable and come in a wide range of colours and styles so you need not look frumpish. They do not have to be dead flat – a small heel is acceptable.

Sore, aching feet

When your feet are tired and sore, they can be revived by soaking them in a footbath of warm water and Epsom salts. This will help ease out any aches and pains and remove the sting and soreness. If you wish, you can buy an electrically powered foot spa-massager which is filled with water and vibrates reassuringly under the feet to reduce any soreness and fatigue. But because the soles are massaged rhythmically it may not work for ticklish feet! Afterwards, dry the feet thoroughly, wiping between the toes and dust with talcum powder or moisturize with some softening cream. Some people think that massaging a little cider vinegar into the soles is invigorating and soothing, too.

Foot problems

Most problems stem from neglect and you must be on the lookout for the warning signs of corns, callouses and the like. Although you can treat some disorders yourself, others require specialist attention from a qualified chiropodist.

1 Corns
These are usually caused by badly fitting shoes which pinch the toes. Sometimes the point of the hard corn that forms on the toe presses inwards on a nerve to cause severe pain. If you see a small newly formed corn, immerse your feet in a warm bath or bowl of water for at least 10 minutes to soften the skin and then rub gently with a pumice stone. You can use a corn plaster to bring relief, but if the corn is deep and really painful it will probably have to be removed professionally.

2 Callouses
Callouses form as patches of hard skin to protect your feet against the damage done by tight shoes. Regular treatment with a pumice stone after soaking the feet in warm water will help remove calloused skin. You can buy a special scraper, too, from most chemists.

3 Athlete's foot
This is a fungus infection which is sometimes picked up at swimming pools, showers, gyms and health clubs. It is easily recognizable as the skin between the toes becomes flaky and dry and later cracked. Exposing the feet so that the air can circulate freely around them helps. Wear sandals in summer or go barefoot at home. You should not wear the same stockings or socks two days running, especially if your feet tend to perspire. Remove any dead skin with a pumice stone, wipe thoroughly dry between the toes and dust with a specially formulated medicated fungicidal powder, or use a cream or lotion available from chemists.

4 Bunions
Although these tend to be regarded as an old person's problem, many young women are affected by them, too. A bunion is a painful swelling at the

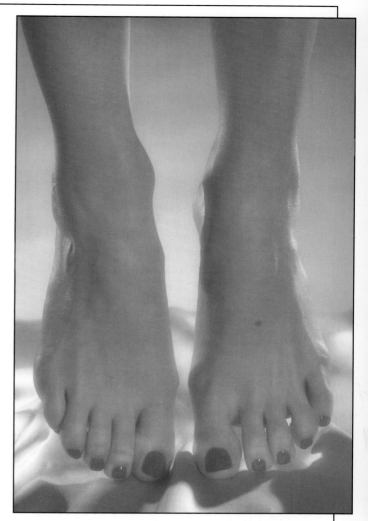

Nail varnishes are available in a wide range of colours. Choose a shade to suit your mood or match your outfit.

side and base of the big toe. It is always caused by tight, badly fitting shoes, so throw out the culprits straight away. There are no home remedies and you should get professional advice as soon as the first signs appear.

Bathtime feet

Use your time in the bath profitably to take care of your feet. Soap them well and then massage gently between fingers and thumbs. Rub away any hard patches of skin with a pumice stone. You can use a loofah to remove any dead skin cells. Brush the nails with a soft nail brush to clean them thoroughly. Afterwards dry well, massage with a moisturizing

Treat your face and feet to a beauty session

hand or body lotion and then lightly dust with talc. Once a week, treat them to a pedicure.

Pedicure

Just as your hands need a weekly manicure beauty treatment, feet need a regular pedicure to keep them smooth, beautiful and free from problems. Try to do it once a week or fortnight, it does not take long and is very comforting and relaxing, too. You will need the same equipment as for your hands – emery boards, creams, varnishes, nail scissors or clippers, cotton wool, orange sticks and a pumice stone.

1 Remove any traces of old nail varnish with polish remover.

2 Soak your feet in a bowl of warm water for 5–10 minutes, adding some Epsom salts if they are feeling tired.

3 Dip them quickly in and out of cold water to stimulate the circulation and prevent nails splitting. Dry thoroughly, especially between the toes which is a good breeding ground for fungus.

4 Trim your nails with scissors or clippers, right back to the end of each toe and cutting straight across – not in a rounded shape. Smooth down any rough edges with an emery board.

5 Dip an orange stick wrapped in a little cotton wool in warm water and gently clean the nails. Apply some cuticle remover and rinse off.

6 Dry and smooth a little cuticle remover into the skin surrounding the nails and the cuticle area.

7 Gently ease back the cuticles with an orange stick.

8 Rinse the feet again in warm water and rub away any patches of hard skin with a pumice stone, or treat with a liquid hard skin remover if persistent.

9 Dry your feet and smooth in some moisturizing hand or body lotion.

10 Separate the toes with cotton wool or sponge pads and apply a base coat of varnish if wished. Allow to dry.

11 Apply a coloured coat of varnish. Dry and apply another coat.

12 When dry apply a protective clear top coat to

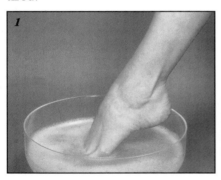

1 For a relaxing pedicure first soak feet in warm water or a foot massager.

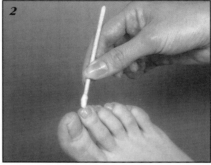

2 Rub cuticle cream into the nails and ease back cuticles with an orange stick.

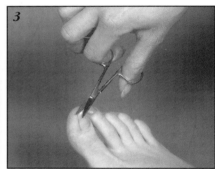

3 Trim nails with clippers or scissors, cutting straight across, not round, the nail.

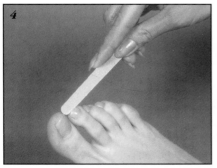

4 File the nails smoothly with an emery board or a file to remove rough edges.

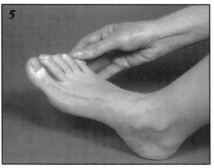

5 Gently massage some moisturizing cream or body lotion into your feet.

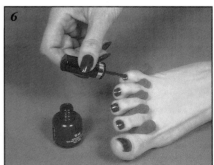

6 Separate your toes with cotton wool and apply two coats of nail polish.

prevent chipping.

13 When dry, dab your feet generously with soothing eau-de-cologne.

Exercises for feet

When you are relaxing at home, it is a good idea to take off your shoes and walk around barefoot to help your feet and toes spread out. Walking and regular foot exercises will boost circulation, strengthen muscles and be surprisingly refreshing. By strengthening your feet you can help ward off fatigue. And because exercise plays an important role in improving circulation, it helps prevent varicose veins and piles, two common pregnancy problems. Here is a simple exercise for you to try:

Foot rotations

Sit on the floor with your left foot under you in a semi-lotus position, with your back straight. Clasp your right knee in your arms and lift your right foot off the ground. Rotate it from the ankle in a large circle through all the points of the compass with your foot flexed. Repeat five times. Then rotate five times with your toes pointed. Repeat with the other leg. You can also do this exercise when sitting at your desk or in a car (as long as you are not driving!) just to boost blood flow to the area. In fact, whenever you sit down for a few minutes, it is a good idea to practise some foot rotations. Another good foot exercise is to practise drawing out the letters of the alphabet in the air with your feet, exaggerating the movements.

Face masks and beauty treatments

Why not treat your skin to a revitalizing face mask this month to pep you up and make you feel marvellous, especially if you are going out on a special date? Face masks can help deep-cleanse the skin, stimulate the circulation and also moisturize and exfoliate. Although they are a marvellous morale booster the effects are only temporary and not long-lasting.

You can buy face masks that are specially formulated for dry or greasy skins as they cleanse deeply, remove excess oil and tighten the pores. They can be easily rinsed off although they look a little frightening on and you should be careful not to surprise anyone or you might give them a nasty shock!

Peel-off masks based on plastic, wax or rubber are best for drier skins. They are gentler than the heavier clay-based sort but not so effective at cleansing. However, when peeled off, some of the dirt and impurities in the skin are removed along with dead skin cells. They soften the skin, leaving it plumped up and pink. These masks evaporate and harden on the skin, constricting the tissues and squeezing the flesh so that you

actually feel your skin tighten and being stretched taut. When the mask is peeled away the skin's blood vessels expand and consequently the skin itself looks fresher, younger and pinker. This is a great lift when you are feeling tired or before an evening out when you want to look your best.

If your skin is oily you should treat yourself to a face mask at least twice a week, whereas dry and normal skins need one only once a week or fortnight. Here's how to apply your face mask:

1 Tie back any strands of hair off the face with pins or a wide-elasticated headband.
2 Deep cleanse your face thoroughly. Rinse with water, dry and tone.
3 When your skin is well-cleansed and dry, smooth in the face mask. Apply it evenly across your face and neck, not too close to the eyes and mouth.
4 Leave the mask on for the recommended time to dry or harden. You can wander around and do things in the meantime; read a book or just lie down with some soothing pads soaked in witch hazel over your eyes.
5 Remove the mask by peeling

off or rinsing clean. Moisturize the skin and look in the mirror. You will be amazed at the difference it has made and how fresh your skin looks and how soft it feels.

Exfoliate your skin

Another way of deep cleansing your skin and removing any waste matter and dead skin cells on the surface is to exfoliate it. You can buy special thinning and abrasive agents for this purpose in the form of gels, creams and lotions which often contain tiny granules. These remove the top layer of cells and stimulate the ones below to leave the skin looking transluscent, smooth and fresh.

After exfoliating, moisturizing will be easier and the creams more readily absorbed by the skin. This is important in pregnancy when your skin may naturally tend to be rather dry and needs deep moisturizing. However, if you are still quite young, say, in your early twenties, it may not be necessary. Women in their thirties will definitely benefit from exfoliation and will be pleased to discover that any tiny fine lines may disappear temporarily afterwards.

Healthy snacks for grazing through the day

This month you may enter what some doctors refer to as the 'grazing stage' of pregnancy, when you feel more comfortable eating smaller, more frequent meals than your normal three a day pattern. This is a good way of avoiding the heartburn that plagues many women during the last trimester. Eating small meals stops you feeling over-full. You must remember that the enlarged uterus leaves less space for your stomach to dilate as it fills the abdominal cavity. This is why you may experience a burning sensation sometimes after eating as food mixed with gastric juices is pushed back up into the oesophagus.

There are ways to avoid this annoying problem and you have to find the method that works best for you. You should not take antacid preparations – natural methods and preventive measures are safer. If you suffer from heartburn, try one of the following:

1 Sip a glass of milk slowly when you begin to feel the telltale signs. This often works and prevents them worsening.

2 Don't eat rich, spicy foods that may irritate your stomach and cause indigestion. Favour milder, plain foods made with simple, wholesome ingredients. Eat slowly – don't gulp your food.

3 After a meal, don't slump down in a chair with the upper part of your uterus resting on your stomach. Instead, sit up straight with a cushion behind your back and wait for your meal to go down and digestion to start.

4 Don't go to bed immediately after eating – stay as upright as possible. If you find it hard to sleep and heartburn occurs, prop yourself up with several cushions or pillows so that you aren't lying flat.

Watch your diet

If eating tends to cause heartburn you may be tempted to skip meals, but it is important for both you and the baby that you continue eating a really healthy diet that supplies all the essential nutrients. Even though your baby is almost fully developed by now, her brain has reached its peak rate of growth, and it is vital to eat a good diet to build new brain

cells. Protein is particularly important, and to be on the safe side you should aim to eat about 75g/3oz daily. Small nutritious snacks of wholemeal bread, cheese, milk, wholewheat biscuits, cold chicken, scrambled eggs, yoghurt or a baked potato with cheese will supply high-quality protein and other nutrients and should not cause heartburn either.

Even if you are alarmed by your fast-growing tummy, you should not try to restrict your calorie intake – you need about 2,400 calories daily to meet your body's own requirements and build your baby's body, too. There is no need to cut down now and prepare for your post-birth figure. Breastfeeding and postnatal exercise will take care of that, and you will soon regain your natural shape if you eat sensibly after your baby is born. As already mentioned, one way not to gain weight in unwanted places, such as hips, arms and thighs, is to stay away from high-calorie foods that lack nutrients like cakes, chocolate, sweets, biscuits, pastries, cream buns and the like.

The grazing stage of pregnancy

Eating high-quality snacks little and often helps you avoid heartburn and this is why some doctors refer to this time as the 'grazing stage' of pregnancy.

Omelettes require little preparation or cooking time and eggs are a good source of protein. Try different fillings and herbs to vary the taste.

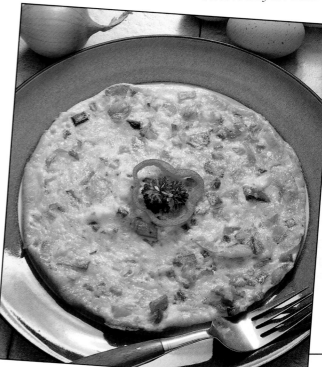

Concentrating on fresh wholesome ingredients of, say, five small meals a day instead of two or three large ones will help reduce heartburn and meet your body's needs. This new style of eating may be necessary for a month or two until your baby's head descends into the pelvis and engages in readiness for labour and birth, and the pressure of the uterus is taken off your stomach.

Here are some ideas and recipes for healthy snacks that are quickly and easily prepared and delicious to eat. They are all nutritious and can be eaten throughout the day. If you are still working, some are suitable for packed lunches and snack boxes to be kept in your desk or in the refrigerator at work for when you need a pick-me-up.

Quick snack meals

All these ideas for snack meals can be quickly prepared – many need no cooking at all. They are nutritious and convenient and should not upset your stomach or cause heartburn.

1   Muesli or granola topped with chopped fruits and yoghurt.
2   Two wholemeal biscuits and a glass of milk.
3   Baked beans on wholemeal toast.
4   Scrambled egg on toast.
5   Sardines on toast – they tend to be oily and the ones canned in tomato sauce may be easier to digest than those in oil.
6   Small pot yoghurt topped with chopped nuts, seeds and wheatgerm.
7   Banana milk shake whizzed up in the blender with whole milk, a ripe banana and yoghurt.
8   Mug of home-made soup – vegetable, lentil, split pea, bean etc.
9   Crudités – carrot and celery sticks; button mushrooms; slices of red and green pepper; cauliflower florets; radishes; cheese cubes; pineapple chunks; olives etc. These can be kept in sealed containers in the refrigerator for appetizing munchies during the day. To keep the vegetables fresh, crisp and moist, stand them in a jug of water. Eat on their own or dipped in yoghurt, mayonnaise, tahini, hummus, mashed avocado, cream cheese etc.
10   Fresh fruit and hunk of cheese.
11   Slice of wholemeal bread spread with honey, pear and apple spread, marmite or peanut butter, and a glass of fruit juice.
12   Small carton of cottage cheese eaten with fruit or raw vegetables.
13   Wholemeal scone and yoghurt.
14   Hard-boiled egg with wholemeal toast.

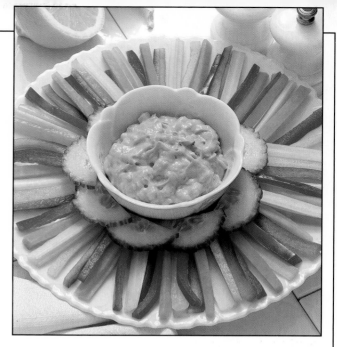

Crudités provide delicious and low-calorie snacks, and for extra taste can be combined with nutritious dips. Whisk up a quick dip with pâté and mushrooms; tomatoes, herbs and ham; or avocado, yoghurt, peppers and lemon juice.

15   Toasted cheese on wholemeal bread topped with sliced avocado.
16   Wholemeal pitta bread filled with salad, cheese, ham, chicken, beans, avocado etc.
17   Half avocado filled with cottage cheese.
18   Two-egg omelette filled with grated cheese, ham, chicken etc.
19   Poached egg on wholemeal toast.
20   Tomato hollowed-out and filled with cottage cheese served with wholemeal bread.

Healthy mini-meals

Again, these meals are easy to put together and do not require long cooking times. Some could be make in large portions and whatever doesn't get eaten can be frozen until a later date. To speed matters up even more, they could be reheated in a microwave oven in just a few minutes.

Healthy beefburgers

Many of the beefburgers you buy in the shops are high in fat and/or cereals. It is best to choose the 100 per cent pure ground beef American sort. However, you can make beefburgers quickly and simply yourself. They are high in protein and are best cooked under a grill rather than fried in hot oil or fat which adds unwanted calories.

Healthy snacks for grazing through the day

175g/6oz very lean ground/minced beef
1 small egg, beaten (or ½ medium to large egg)
1 small onion, finely chopped
few drops Worcestershire sauce
2 round wholemeal rolls or baps
tomato sauce (see recipe)
mustard
lettuce leaves (optional)

Mix the beef, beaten egg and onion. Season with salt and pepper and the Worcestershire sauce. Form the mixture into two smooth patties. Place under a hot grill and when one side is browned and cooked, turn over and cook the other side. Pop into the split rolls and top with tomato sauce and mustard. Add some shredded lettuce if wished; or a slice of Swiss cheese, and pop back under the grill until melted before replacing the top half of the roll.

Jacket baked potato
One of the healthiest and easiest mini-meals of all, a baked potato retains its vitamin C and is high in protein, too. Topping it with cheese, ham, chicken or prawns will increase the grams of protein even more. This is not suitable for freezing.

1 large baking potato

Scrub the potato well and cut out any blemishes. Pierce the skin with a sharp skewer or fork, and bake in a preheated oven at 200°C, 400°F, gas 6 for about 1 hour. The outer case should be slightly crisp and the insides soft. Top or stuff as suggested below:
1   Split and top with soured cream or *fromage frais* and chopped chives. Sprinkle with plenty of freshly ground black pepper and season with sea salt.
2   Scoop out the insides and mix with 25g/1oz each cream cheese and peeled prawns and a few chopped chives or parsley stalks.
3   Scoop out the insides and mix with 45ml/3 tablespoons cottage cheese, 1 chopped spring onion and a little chopped pineapple.
4   Scoop out the insides and mix with 25g/1oz

crumbled blue cheese, 2 crumbled grilled bacon rashers (or equivalent ham, chopped) and top with soured cream and chives.
5   Top with 25g/1oz baked beans and diced ham.
6   Top with 30ml/2 tablespoons cottage cheese, a slice of raw mushroom and cress.
7   Top with smoked Continental sausage and parsley.
8   Top with 3 rolls of salami and a spoonful of cucumber relish.
9   Top with coleslaw or salad vinaigrette and a sprig of watercress.
10   Top with 4 peeled prawns and some sautéed peppers and onions.

Brown rice savoury
Brown rice is a good source of fibre in your diet, and also contains protein and B vitamins. This is easy to make but is not suitable for freezing.

50g/2oz/¼ cup long-grain brown rice
small knob butter
25g/1oz/¼ cup walnuts, chopped
1 tomato, skinned and sliced
25g/1oz/⅛ cup currants or raisins
1 spring onion, chopped
few drops soya sauce
salt and pepper
30ml/2 tablespoons grated Cheddar cheese

Cook the rice until tender in salted boiling water (or stock for a better, more savoury flavour). Drain and gently mix in the butter, nuts, tomato, currants, onion and soya sauce. Check the seasoning. Sprinkle with grated cheese and put in a warm oven to heat through, until the cheese melts. Serve immediately, with a green or orange salad if wished.

Healthy hot dogs
Do not be tempted to use ordinary frankfurters in this recipe – they are crammed full of additives and are far from healthy. Some butchers make their own additive-free sausages often seasoned with spices or herbs, and these are the best sort to use. Of course, you can make your own sausages but this is time-consuming and most of us cannot be bothered.

1 large sausage
1 long wholemeal roll
tomato sauce (see recipe)

mustard
lettuce leaves (optional)

Grill the sausage until well-browned and cook right through, turning occasionally. Split a wholemeal roll and place the sausage inside. Dribble over some hot tomato sauce (you can use ketchup although the flavour is not so good) and a little mustard. For extra interest, add a few chopped lettuce leaves if wished and sandwich together.

Pitta bread pizza

This is so quick to make and the wholemeal pitta base saves you the tedium of making bread dough. Again, it is not suitable for freezing and should be eaten immediately.

1 wholemeal pitta bread
30-45ml/2-3 tablespoons tomato sauce
(recipe below)
50g/2oz chopped ham or shrimps
sprinkling oregano or basil
3 slices Mozzarella cheese
2 anchovy fillets (optional)
2 black olives
trickle of olive oil

Top the pitta bread with the tomato sauce, ham or shrimps (or sliced fried mushrooms if you prefer) and sprinkle with herbs. Cover with cheese and the anchovies and olives. Brush with oil if wished to keep the topping moist. Place on a baking sheet under a hot grill for about 10 minutes, or in a preheated oven at 200°C, 400°F, gas 6 for 15 minutes until golden and cooked. Serve with salad.

Tomato sauce

This recipe makes several servings – more than you will need for one pitta bread pizza. It can also be used to top spaghetti or may be served with beefburgers, sausages, baked potatoes or cauliflower. Freeze until required in individual portions.

1 small onion, chopped
15ml/1 tablespoon oil
450g/1lb tomatoes, skinned and chopped or
400g/14oz canned tomatoes
pinch brown sugar
5ml/1 teaspoon tomato paste

2.5ml/½ teaspoon mixed herbs
salt and pepper

Fry the onion gently in the oil until tender. Add the remaining ingredients and cook over medium heat for 10-15 minutes until the sauce is thick and reduced.

Mini quiches

This recipe makes four mini-quiches. Freeze what you do not eat, or put one aside in the refrigerator until tomorrow. A quiche makes a convenient nutritious meal – quite light when you don't feel like a big meal. The wholemeal flour, eggs and milk make it a good source of protein, and you can fill it with the flavouring ingredients of your choice. Make the quiches up in little pie tins or aluminium foil mini-containers. For speed and ease make the pastry in a food processor rather than by hand.

Pastry:
100g/4oz/½ cup vegetable margarine
225g/8oz/2¼ cups wholemeal flour
pinch salt
45ml/3 tablespoons cold water
Filling:
3 medium eggs
200ml/8floz/1 cup milk
salt and pepper
pinch ground nutmeg
45ml/3 tablespoons cream (optional)
50g/2oz/½ cup grated cheese
Flavourings, choose one of the following:
3 leeks, sliced and sautéed; 3 sliced skinned tomatoes and 4 black olives or
675g/1½lb spinach, chopped and cooked; 100g/4oz streaky bacon and 1 chopped onion, sautéed or
100g/4oz flaked cooked smoked haddock

Make the pastry: either make up in the food processor or rub the fat into the flour and salt. Add the water and mix to a soft dough. Rest in the refrigerator for 10-15 minutes before rolling out and lining 4 small tins.

Make the filling: beat the eggs, milk and seasoning, adding the cream if used. Mix with the flavouring of your choice and pour into the prepared tins. Sprinkle with cheese and bake in a preheated oven at 200°C, 400°F, gas 6 for 15 minutes. Lower the temperature to 180°C, 350°F, gas 4 and bake for a further 20 minutes until set and golden-brown.

EXERCISE 7

Watch your posture and avoid backache

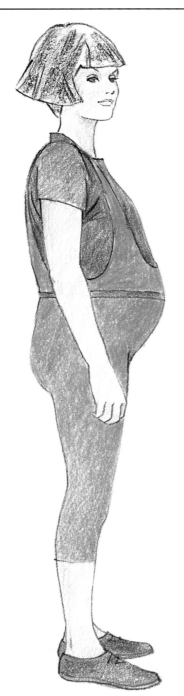

Good posture is very important in pregnancy, especially in the later months when your 'bump' gets larger and you may suffer from annoying backache. If you walk, stand and sit correctly, you will not only feel better and more comfortable but you are also more likely to regain your figure easily after the baby is born. This is because your spine and abdominal muscles will be stronger. Simple exercises will soon firm them up and get you back into shape.

So why do so many pregnant women have debilitating backache as a result of bad posture? Well, there are two main reasons:

1   During the last three months, the ligaments supporting the spine are softened by extra progesterone in your body.

2   As your abdomen gets progressively larger, your centre of gravity shifts forwards in front of your pelvis. Half the weight you put on in pregnancy is concentrated in this area and to counteract this, many women tend to throw their shoulders back and thrust their stomach outwards creating a hollow in the lower back. This does not distribute the weight of the back evenly and puts more strain on the spine and back joints. Far from alleviating the problem it will make any backache even worse.

Good posture

The secret of good posture is to adjust it as the weight load of the baby increases. You must be well balanced with the baby's weight distributed evenly across your body so as to reduce the strain on muscles and joints and make you feel more comfortable.

Check your natural posture by standing sideways in front of a full length mirror and examine your profile. Ask yourself the following questions and answer them honestly:

1   Are you holding your shoulders too high? They should be dropped and easy to keep your spine straight and ease out any tension. Never fling them back like a guardsman standing to attention on parade.

2   Is the curve at the back of your waist over-exaggerated? It should be fairly straight and not indented or hollow as this allows your abdominal muscles to sag and distorts your spine. It also puts increased pressure on the lower back and causes a

Good posture is essential as your baby gets heavier. Stand straight with your shoulders dropped and relaxed, your chest high and your buttocks and stomach pulled in.

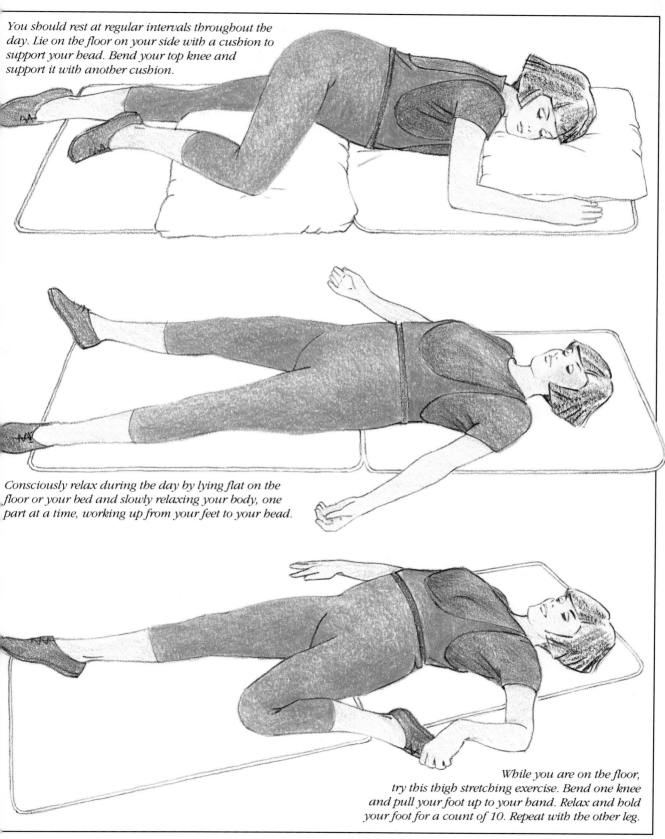

You should rest at regular intervals throughout the day. Lie on the floor on your side with a cushion to support your head. Bend your top knee and support it with another cushion.

Consciously relax during the day by lying flat on the floor or your bed and slowly relaxing your body, one part at a time, working up from your feet to your head.

While you are on the floor, try this thigh stretching exercise. Bend one knee and pull your foot up to your hand. Relax and hold your foot for a count of 10. Repeat with the other leg.

Watch your posture and avoid backache

great deal of backache which is avoidable.

3 Are your ribs and chest high enough? They should be lifted so that you have sufficient space to breathe.

To improve your posture you should try standing with your back against a wall, your shoulders and bottom only in contact with it. Now, keeping your shoulders dropped and relaxed, press the small of your back into the wall. At the same time, imagine that your head is being pulled upwards and stand up tall. Walk away from the wall in this posture. Try not to be stiff and awkward – let your muscles relax and feel comfortable. Remember to keep your shoulders dropped and your buttocks tucked in, and you should feel well-balanced and easy without a trace of tension.

Try to be aware of your posture at all times and correct it immediately if you feel yourself throwing your weight forwards and the tell-tale hollow in your back becomes more exaggerated. When you stand still, you should also try to distribute the extra weight evenly. The best way to do this is to stand up tall with your feet square – don't shift your weight backwards and forwards between your feet or favour one leg and rest your weight on that.

Sit up straight

You may be tired and there is a great temptation to slump forwards in a chair at an awkward angle but this is the worst thing you can possibly do for you back. If you want to avoid backache, especially in the lower lumbar region, you must always sit tall with your spine well supported. If you slump or let your upper body rest on your abdomen, you are effectively leaning on your uterus and putting additional strain on your poor stomach and liver.

It is very important to have a well-designed, comfortable chair, and you should ensure that the chair you sit on at the office or at home and also your car seat have adequate lumbar support for your spine. If necessary, place a cushion strategically behind you to support the small of your back, especially if you are sitting at a desk working or

typing for long periods. Sit well back on the chair, not on the edge, with your thighs, pelvis and spine supported. Make sure also that the seat does not press into the backs of your legs, nor should you cross them – this can interfere with circulation and contribute to the formation of ugly varicose veins.

If your back starts to ache, when you have been sitting at a desk working for a long time, lower your head and rest it on the table in front of you. This will help ease out your spine and stretch out the back of your neck, relieving any tension in this region.

Bending and lifting

When you are pregnant, you must learn how to bend over, lift and carry heavy objects without putting additional strain on your back and abdominal muscles. The golden rule to remember is *never* to lean over from the waist to pick anything up. And this should apply to everybody at all times – not just when you are pregnant. If we all treated our backs with respect and bent down properly we would avoid a lot of unnecessary backache.

When you want to pick anything up from a lower level or from the floor, bend your knees and gently lower yourself into a squatting position. Keep your back straight and let your legs take the strain. As you rise, hold the object close to your body and continue to keep your spine straight. Brace your thighs and straighten your knees as you push your feet against the floor. Be sure not to rise at an angle or twist awkwardly. Kneel or squat when making beds, cleaning baths and doing other household tasks – *don't* bend over. When cleaning floors, use a long-handled mop or get down on all-fours. Surprisingly, many doctors recommend this position (and activity!) for the relief of backache, as it takes the weight of the baby off the spine.

When carrying heavy bags such as shopping, make sure that you are evenly balanced on both sides. Never put all the shopping into one basket – better to divide it between two and carry two equal weights. If possible, avoid carrying heavy things altogether. Supermarket shopping is easy if you can load the bags into a trolley and push it out to the car to unload. Better still, take your partner with you and let him be your packhorse.

Exercises for relieving backache

These simple exercises help relieve back pains and strengthen the spine. Practise them every day:

1 Angry cat
This is a yoga posture which is particularly useful during pregnancy, and helps relieve tired, aching back muscles. Kneel on the floor with your arms and legs in line supporting your weight evenly. Make sure that your back is straight and not sagging in the middle. You will feel more comfortable immediately as the weight of the baby is taken off your spine. Now raise your back slowly and drop your head and shoulders. Exhale as you do so and tighten your stomach muscles and buttocks and pull in your pelvic floor muscles. Inhale deeply and slowly and then relax into the starting position with your back flat. Repeat this exercise 5 times each day.

2 Shoulder rolls
If you get upper backache and tension between the shoulder blades the worst thing you can do to ease it is to fling your shoulders back and tighten the muscles in the upper back. Many women tend to do this unconsciously to compensate for the extra weight. Shoulder rolls are a good way of relieving this upper back pain. Their great advantage is that they can be done anywhere – at your desk, in a bus queue or sitting at home. All you do is to sit on a chair with your back straight and rest your fingertips on your shoulders – right hand on right shoulder and left hand on left shoulder. Now rotate your elbows slowly backwards, rolling the whole upper arm from the shoulder. Repeat the exercise about 10 times until the pain eases out.

3 Tailor sitting
You can lengthen and stretch your spine by sitting cross-legged against a wall. If you are sitting correctly, you should be able to feel the whole length of your spine against the wall. If you can only feel part of it, then it's too rounded. Draw in your legs close to your body and sit cross-legged. You will be surprised at how comfortable you feel. This position prevents the weight of the uterus resting on the upper thighs and blocking circulation to your lower legs. It also brings hips level with feet to enhance blood flow in the area – another way of helping prevent varicose veins. Sit like this to read a book or watch TV. You do not need a wall for support as you get used to tailor sitting, but do not slouch.

4 Bridging
Backache may also be caused by weak abdominal muscles – you can straighten them with bridging exercises. These bring other benefits, too, as they tighten up buttock muscles and improve circulation in the legs. Lie on the floor with your head resting on a comfortable cushion, arms at your sides and your legs raised, heels resting on a low stool or table. Now tighten your abdominal and buttock muscles as you raise your buttocks off the floor. Be sure to keep your back straight. Hold the position for a count of 5 and then slowly lower your bottom to the floor. Repeat 5 times. This exercise sounds more difficult than it really is. You will discover that it is quite gentle and easy to perform.

5 Tummy strengthener
Lie on a mat or towel on the floor with some cushions to support your head and shoulders. Bend your knees with your feet flat on the floor about shoulder width apart. Lift your head and shoulders slightly off the floor and extend your left hand out to touch your right knee. Lower yourself to the floor without touching down with your head and repeat to the other side, touching your left knee with your right hand. Repeat 10 times on each side. If you feel any pain or strain in the abdominal area when performing these exercises, stop at once.

Avoiding backache

Practise good posture, lift and carry objects correctly and perform the exercises outlined above and you will go a long way towards avoiding backache. Of course, in the very last month, some backache is inevitable due to hormonal changes as your body prepares itself for the delivery and loosens up accordingly. Also, the fitter, stronger and more flexible you are, the better your chances of avoiding backache. So regular exercise will help as it strengthens muscles, prevents you putting on excess weight which may put additional strain on the spine, and keeps you generally feeling better and looking good.

Remember that good posture improves your appearance in addition to solving back problems. If you walk tall and gracefully, you will look slimmer and healthier and feel more comfortable. People you meet will congratulate you on how well you look.

And if you do get backache . . . Well, try the exercises, especially the angry cat pose. Lie down and relax with your back well-supported. Sleep on a firm, not a soft, mattress. Or relax in a soothing bath to ease out tension – try adding some fragrant oil or herbs to the water to make it more luxurious and enjoyable.

How to stay healthy in the final months

If you are still working, you may be advised by your doctor, family and friends to slow down or stop now. In this last trimester of your pregnancy, you will feel increasingly heavy and slow and you do need to put aside time every day for rest and relaxation. However, it is perfectly possible to work right up to the day labour starts – it all depends on your level of health and fitness. You are the best judge of whether you should continue working and for how long.

However, if you are continually tired, tense and under stress in your job, you would be well advised to stop or to work part-time instead. Your doctor may give you a kick chart so that you can record the movements of your baby in the womb. Some women who work say that they do not feel their babies moving regularly throughout the day – only in the evenings when they relax and put their feet up. It may be that they are too busy to notice any movements or that their babies are rocked to sleep by their being on the move.

A kick chart is a means of checking on your baby and her wellbeing. All you have to do is to shade a square according to when you feel your baby move. You will probably be advised to contact the hospital if you feel no movements at all in a 12-hour period. You may need to have your baby's heartbeat monitored – an easy and totally painless procedure. Of course, if you are working hard or extremely busy, it may be the case that if you slow down and sit down, that you will soon feel a movement. Many women find that their babies are most active when they go to bed at night!

Toxaemia

This disorder may happen in late pregnancy – it affects between five and ten per cent of pregnant women. The warning signs are:

- raised blood pressure
- headaches and dizziness
- excessive swelling (oedema) in the ankles and fingers
- anaemia

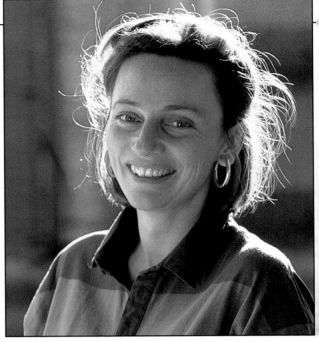

You can stay healthy and fit in the final trimester of your pregnancy if you continue to eat sensibly and rest every day. Try to practise your relaxation exercises regularly.

- protein in the urine
- high weight gain.

Your doctor will watch out for any of these signs as your pregnancy progresses. When you visit your surgery or clinic, you will always be weighed, your blood pressure taken, your ankles examined and your urine tested.

So what is toxaemia? It is the reason for many stillbirths, infant deaths and 50 per cent of low birth weight, premature babies. It may also cause the mother's liver to malfunction.

How can it be avoided? The best way to prevent toxaemia (and the easiest) is to eat a really healthy diet which supplies all the nutrients that both you and your baby need for optimum health. Malnourished women who eat nutritionally poor foods with a high percentage of over-refined processed products, may be deficient in essential protein, minerals (like magnesium), vitamins, especially folic acid (liver and dark green leafy vegetables) and vitamin B6. Eating a good diet and preventing toxaemia is not necessarily linked to social class or income level. During both world wars when food rationing was enforced in Britain, and sugar, white flour and processed nutritionally poor foods were not available, the incidence of toxaemia fell drastically. Consequently, healthier babies were born to women who ate more fibre and whole-grain cereals, vegetables and pulses and less fat and sugar.

Do not worry unduly if you have slight swelling, sudden weight gain or the occasional headache – these can all be perfectly normal and are not necessarily symptoms of toxaemia. If you are worried, you should consult your doctor. However, a few doctors who are worried about the possibility of toxaemia, may tell women to restrict their calorie intake, opt for a low-sodium (low-salt) diet and use diuretics to minimize fluid retention. Far from reducing the risk of toxaemia, these measures may have the opposite effect to that intended and actually increase the possibility since blood volume may fall and affect the kidneys.

Of course, it is sensible from a health and beauty point of view not to gain excessive weight – say, not more than 30lb. However, if you deliberately restrict your weight gain with the result that you are underweight and malnourished, you are potentially a more likely target for toxaemia. By eating a healthy varied diet along the lines laid down in the diet sections of this book, you can ensure that you have a happy, trouble-free pregnancy and a healthy baby.

Fluid retention

This is very common in the last two or three months. Some swelling is not abnormal during pregnancy as your body gets ready for labour and breastfeeding by storing fluids to prevent dehydration. This swelling quickly subsides after birth as you eliminate excess fluid. So you can see that a small increase in fluid is actually protective rather than hazardous as it ensures a reserve for your expanding blood volume as the placenta grows, *and* adequate flow of milk for your baby after birth.

But if you eat a poor diet and receive insufficient nutrients for producing albumin in your liver, any swelling can be potentially hazardous. You need some albumin circulating in your bloodstream to draw water into circulation and attract the fluid-carrying waste products from the cells for excretion by the kidneys. But if the albumin levels are low, water may leak from the blood vessels into the tissues and cause them to swell. Your kidneys may fail to excrete wastes efficiently from your body and this, in turn, can affect the normal functioning of the placenta. The recognizable symptoms are puffy, swollen skin, especially on your face, swollen ankles and difficulty removing your rings at night.

Some women try to counter this by reducing the amount of fluid they drink, but this is not a good thing. You must try to eat an adequate amount of protein each day to help maintain albumin levels in your bloodstream. This will stop excessive swelling. On no account, should you take diuretics or 'water' tablets, or restrict your salt intake. Both these actions could be potentially harmful to your baby.

You may be surprised to learn that some salt is necessary for maintaining good health. Although limiting salt intake can reduce the amount of water held in the tissues, it also restricts the normal expansion of blood volume which is vital for the health and growth of the placenta. Studies have shown that women who salt their food to taste and do not attempt to restrict their intake, have less muscle cramps, a lower incidence of toxaemia and swelling. They also have fewer birth complications, premature births and haemorrhages. Yet despite the mass of evidence now available, there are still a few doctors who continue to put pregnant women on low-sodium diets.

Diuretics may also be prescribed to deal with fluid retention, but although they reduce the amount of waste in the tissues, they also decrease your blood volume. And when you excrete large amounts of water from the body, you lose water-soluble vitamins, too. Body fluids may be forced so rapidly through the kidneys that any nutrients therein cannot be absorbed into your bloodstream in time.

Try to improve the quality of your diet rather than take diuretics. If you are getting enough protein and vitamin B6 for its metabolism, you are unlikely to suffer from excessive swelling. Of course, even on the healthiest diet, your feet and ankles may swell a little from the weight of the uterus pressing on the veins that transport blood back to your heart from the legs. This may cause pooling of fluid in your lower legs so that you should lie down with a pillow under your head and your feet and legs elevated above you, either resting on a chair, stool or low table, or up against a wall. This position enables your blood to return to the heart.

Remember that ankles and feet can swell more in hot weather or if you have been standing still for some time – just elevate your legs and the swelling should subside. Never sit with your legs crossed or the chair seat pressing into them as this can restrict blood flow, too. Rotate your ankles regularly and practise drawing patterns and words in the air with each foot to promote better circulation. Sitting cross-legged may also help as this brings your feet level with your hips and prevents any pooling of blood and fluids.

Your baby 'engages' ready for labour

You

Only two more months to go now, and you are probably very relieved that the delivery date is drawing nearer as you feel progressively heavier. Of course, not all women feel uncomfortable or slowed down by their pregnancy at this stage. If you are one of this fortunate band, you should still try to make an effort to rest for an hour or two every day and put your feet up even if you feel perfectly fit and active.

Your baby is probably moving a lot now and whenever you sit down or go to bed, you become very aware of her movements and kicks. Soon you will become conscious, too, of the so-called Braxton-Hicks contractions which are preparing your uterus for labour. During one of these contractions, you may feel slight discomfort, and if you place one hand on your abdomen you will feel it hardening as the uterus contracts. These will get stronger in the last weeks.

You may find that your doctor or clinic now requires you to make regular weekly visits for check-ups – just to ensure that your pregnancy is progressing normally, that you are well and the baby is healthy. This is the month when the baby spins round to 'present' herself for labour – this usually happens around the thirty-second week in first pregnancies, and a little later, the thirty-fourth week, in subsequent ones. During check-ups, your midwife or doctor will check on the baby's presentation, and may even try to turn her if she takes her time and is still in the breech position. This is nothing to worry about and does not hurt. A skilled doctor can turn a baby by pressing his hands gently but firmly on your abdomen. Despite

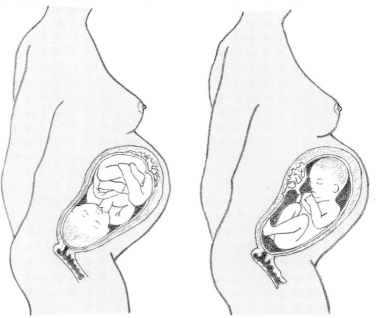

this, a lot of stubborn babies turn back round again afterwards! If turning does not work and the baby is a breech birth, you should not be unduly alarmed. Talk the situation over with your doctor and midwife and see what they advise. A lot of breech babies can still be delivered vaginally without recourse to a Caesarian section. Even then, it is a safe procedure and may be performed with you fully conscious under epidural anaesthesia.

Your baby

By the eighth month, your baby is about 40cm/16in long and fully formed. During the course of the next four weeks she will grow at least 5cm/2in in length and put on weight, too, as she continues to lay down fat reserves in preparation for birth. All she needs now is another layer of insulating fat and some lung surfactant.

Even in the cosy, dark womb, she is aware of some external stimuli and phenomena. For example, she may move about and kick her legs when she hears music – for this reason, many mothers play tapes of soothing light or classical music to their unborn children. Your baby can even distinguish between light and dark, and if you sunbathe, she will be aware of a reddish glow.

When your baby presents herself, it may be backwards or forwards. In the anterior position the baby lies with her back against the mother's abdomen, whereas in the posterior position, her back is next to your spine. Because she can lie to the right or left, her position will be referred to as right or left anterior or right or left posterior. The baby has now filled nearly all the available space in the uterus and she will turn her feet slightly inwards with both legs bent at the hips and knees and crossed. Her arms cross, too, with the right hand resting on the left shoulder and vice versa. Usually her chin rests on her chest with her head and neck bent forwards.

If your baby was born at the end of the eighth month in the thirty-sixth week, she would have a ninety per cent chance of survival. From now onwards, through the last month of your pregnancy, she will gain about 28g/1oz every day so it is important that you should continue eating a healthy diet and not start cutting back on food due to heartburn, tiredness or even a desire to regain your pre-pregnancy figure more quickly after birth.

The illustrations (left) show the cephalic and breech presentations. The baby on the far left is a normal cephalic presentation whereas the one on the near left is in the breech position. There is still plenty of time for your baby to turn, but your consultant may still suggest turning her manually or even book you in for a Caesarean section. Talk over the various options and his/her reasons for the suggested course of action before agreeing or making up your own mind.

Go on a shopping spree

Now is the time to go out shopping and stock up on food for your larder and freezer, or buy baby clothes and equipment, and any essential items you may need for your confinement such as a new nightdress, gown or slippers. Babies can come early and it is best to be ready and not caught out by a sudden arrival. From the end of this month, your overnight bag should be packed in readiness for a quick get-away at whatever time of day or night. Also, you may not feel like long shopping trips next month if you get even heavier and slower so do it now. You may even wish to decorate the baby's room and make it look pretty for its new occupant. However, get your partner or friend to help you and do not climb ladders or over-tire yourself. Bear in mind that babies seem to like bright, cheerful, primary colours rather than pastel shades. The baby will need a cot or crib possibly with a mobile suspended above it, a changing mat and a chest of drawers for her clothes. It is useful also to put a comfortable chair in her room if you intend to breastfeed her.

Revitalize your skin and create a party face

When you are feeling tired or heavy during the last month or two of your pregnancy and can hardly wait for the baby to be born, it is sometimes hard to take the time and trouble to stay beautiful. A lot of women feel washed-out and drained of energy and consequently cannot be bothered to apply any make-up or wash their hair as regularly as usual. But the better you look the better you will feel as a result, and it is important not to neglect your beauty routines now. You are experiencing a very special beauty and can still glow outwardly and radiate health and happiness.

Of course, not all women feel like this – some continue to be energetic and don't seem to suffer from any pregnancy-related aches and pains. They can work right up to the day they give birth without feeling even a twinge of backache! Often, these women take more care of themselves and their appearance than their sisters who stay at home. Perhaps this is because waiting passively rarely brings fulfillment and can be tedious and boring. However, if you do work, you must be sure to make time to rest every day and not to overdo it.

To help ensure that your skin stays clear and glowing, try to cleanse, tone and moisturize in the mornings, evenings and before applying make-up.

Fatigue and your skin

Your skin is an effective barometer of how you feel and if you are tired it will soon show in your face – you may look pale and washed-out; your skin sallow and grey. If you aren't getting enough sleep, tell-tale dark rings may appear under your eyes. However, you *can* still look good. The first step is to try to get some more rest and sleep. If you sleep badly at night, try supplementing these hours with a nap during the day. Make the bed as comfortable as possible with cushions and a backrest, and don't forget to tuck a soft pillow under your 'bump' to bring relief.

Disguise dark shadows under the eyes with some concealer. Dot it onto the skin and gently smooth in. Don't pull the delicate tissue around the eyes. Now apply your foundation evenly to give a healthy look, add colour and even out skin tone, making your skin look soft and smooth. Choose a shade that is only one or two tones darker than your natural skin tone so that it does not create an unnatural effect. In summer, you can use a moisturizing bronze gel to give a natural-looking tanned appearance. Of course, if it is hot and sunny, you may develop a tan anyway and this always helps promote a picture of health and disguises any fatigue that you may be feeling.

By using blusher cleverly you can add much-needed colour and make your face come alive. It will also help define your cheekbones and give shape and definition to your face. Never apply bright red spots of colour that stand out unnaturally against your normal skin tone. The secret is to blend the blusher lightly along the cheekbones for a more natural effect. Bright clear roses, pinks and apricots are best for daytime – not muddy browns,

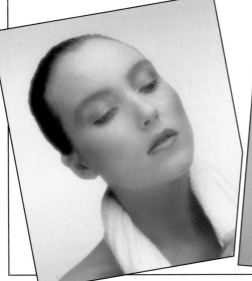
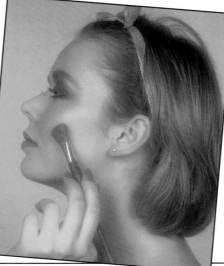

Use a concealer liquid or stick around your mouth, nose and under your eyes, to hide blemishes and shadows and even out your features. After applying a smooth layer of foundation, remove any areas of shine with powder. Then define and highlight your cheek-bones with a subtle shade of blusher.

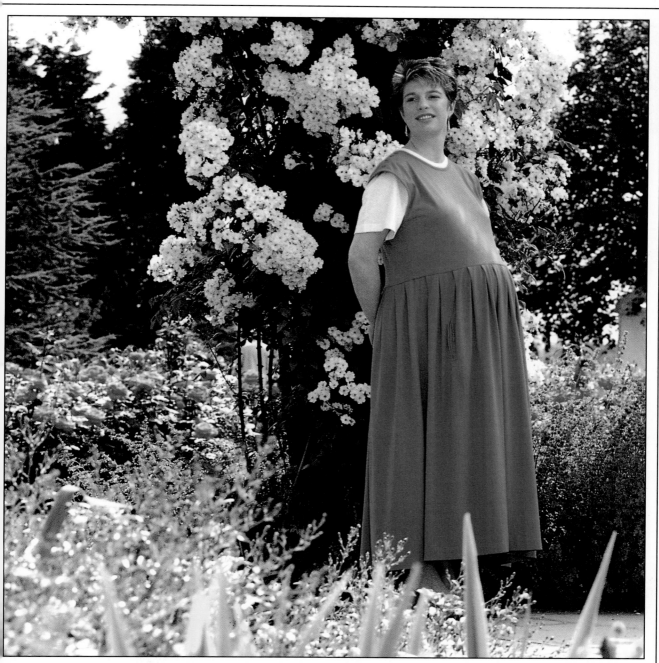

terracottas, bright reds and fuchsias which are better reserved for evening wear. You will probably find that a light powder is best as it does not smudge or block the pores. Some creams and gels can feel slightly greasy on the skin.

Puffy eyes, hands and feet

Puffy eyes can be a sign of tiredness or a result of fluid retention which is a common problem in the eighth and ninth months for many women. If your eyes look sore and swollen, the best remedy is to soak two cotton wool balls in some witch hazel, squeeze out and place one over each eye. A cold flannel can also work wonders if you haven't any witch hazel handy. To try and combat fluid retention you should drink plenty of mineral water and avoid eating highly salted foods. Elevating your legs and feet at regular intervals throughout the day will help

Revitalize your skin and create a party face

prevent swollen ankles and feet, as will light exercise and sitting cross-legged so that your feet and legs are level with your hips.

Don't be alarmed if you experience slight swelling – some is perfectly normal as your body actually stores fluids to prevent dehydration as it prepares itself for labour and breastfeeding. So some fluid is really a kind of protective mechanism to ensure a reserve for your expanding blood volume as the placenta grows. However, if you are not eating a nutritious healthy diet, excessive swelling may sometimes be hazardous – your doctor, midwife or clinic will keep an eye on this when you make your usual visits, especially in the last few weeks.

The nutrients you get from the food you eat help produce albumin in your liver. Its function is to draw water into circulation and thus attract the fluid carrying waste products from the cells for excretion by the kidneys. When albumin levels are low, water sometimes leaks from the blood vessels into the surrounding tissues and makes them swell. Your face may look swollen, your skin puffy and you may experience difficulties removing your rings at night.

Many women mistakenly think that cutting down on the amount of fluid they drink will combat the swelling but this is not true. The most important thing is to make sure that you are eating an adequate amount of protein to help maintain sufficient albumin in your bloodstream to stop any swelling becoming serious. You need about 75g/3oz protein daily for your health and that of your baby. Your doctor may even advise you to restrict your salt intake or take diuretics to reduce the swelling. Talk it over together first as recent research has shown that both these measures may be potentially hazardous to the baby. You need some salt for the maintenance of good health, the normal expansion of blood volume in your body and the growth of the placenta. In experiments when women were encouraged to salt their food to taste and not to restrict their intake, they experienced fewer muscle cramps, a lower incidence of swelling and less birth complications than women who restricted their intake.

Of course, however healthy your diet, you may sometimes experience some swelling, especially in the feet and ankles, just from the weight of the uterus pressing on the veins that carry blood back to your heart from the lower legs. If this is the case, lie down with your legs elevated above you on a stool, low table or against the wall. Don't sit with your legs crossed or with a hard seat pressing into the back of them – this can also restrict blood flow and contribute to swelling. Practise your ankle rotations regularly.

Dealing with dry skin

When your abdomen gets large with the growing baby, your skin will be stretched taut and may be very dry and rather itchy. Resist the temptation to scratch, and attack the condition instead. Daily bathing will help if you add a few drops of soothing, moisturizing oil to the water. Don't use soap as this only makes the dryness worse. Afterwards, smooth in a softening cream or body lotion – baby oil is especially effective as a lubricant for the dry skin on the abdomen, breasts and thighs. Although it may not prevent stretch marks it will keep the skin feeling soft and smooth and avoid any irritating itching.

Condition your hair

As I've already stated, it is all too easy to neglect yourself during these uncomfortable last weeks. Your hair, in particular, may become dry and out of condition. To keep it glossy, healthy-looking and soft, it needs regular care and attention. It is sometimes hard to summon up the energy to shampoo it when it means leaning over a sink with your 'bump' getting in the way. If you experience difficulties washing your hair, try doing it in the bath or shower instead which may prove more comfortable.

A good conditioner will help protect your hair by sealing the hair shafts, filling in any splits and giving it a smooth surface. Instant creme conditioning rinses cannot repair hair damage but merely mask any faults on a temporary basis. To restore health, shine and bounce to dry hair and make it more manageable and less flyaway, you need a deep-conditioning treatment that penetrates right down to the inner cortex of each hair and actually bonds and strengthens it. A protein treatment pack is very effective and will help restore strength and suppleness to minimize the damage.

Oil and wax treatments are also good for treating dry, lifeless hair. Although they take time to apply and act, they really do nourish the hair and leave it looking glossy. Henna conditioning wax, made from the leaves of old plants that have lost their colouring properties, is very effective. Like a hot oil treatment, it is applied to the hair after shampooing and rinsing and then the head is wrapped in a warm, damp towel for a specified amount of time. Used once a week, it will help protect your hair and keep it shiny, silky and glossy. You will also find that tangles may become a thing of the past.

Evening glamour

Just because you're eight months pregnant does not mean that you have to sit quietly at home watching TV every evening or go into seclusion. You can still go out and enjoy yourself *and* look good even though you may feel large or slightly uncomfortable. There are some very flattering maternity dresses and trouser suits or silky jumpsuits when you feel like dressing up. And you can transform your daytime make-up into a party look with added glitter, glosses and brighter shimmering colours.

Obviously, don't overdo it and literally dance the night away if you are feeling tired or run-down – you need your sleep more than ever now. When you're seated, make sure that your back is well supported and avoid any cigarettes or alcohol that may be offered. Nobody is going to be offended if you stick to mineral water, fruit juices or soft drinks. Wear low shoes in a pretty colour which do not pinch your feet, especially if you are dancing. Don't indulge in any vigorous disco routines – stick to gentle movements and romantic dances in your partner's arms!

Make-up: as we have already seen, make-up can improve on nature, enhance your natural good features and cover any blemishes. When you go out for an evening, make the effort to look suitably glamorous with some dazzling make-up. It will make you feel good.

1 Apply your usual foundation or tinted moisturizer.

2 Dot concealer under tired eyes and over any spots or blemishes.

3 Define your cheekbones with a shimmering blusher – try a dusting of silky powder or some shiny cheek gloss.

4 If you are skilful, apply some highlighters under the brows and blend with a clean brush for subtle shine.

5 Outline your eyes with eyeliner or a soft smoky pencil. For evenings, you can forget the boring old browns and greys, and try an iridescent brilliant blue, bright green or violet instead.

6 Now apply eye shadow to match or complement your pencil colour. Use a darker shade in the socket and a lighter shade on the eyelid itself.

7 Mascara your lashes, top and bottom. If it does not irritate your eyes, use a lash thickener for a really luxuriant effect, perhaps in a dazzling blue or green for a party look.

8 If wished, set your make-up with some translucent powder for a really smooth finish that will not streak under hot lights or in a warm atmosphere.

9 Apply a bright lipstick, outlining your lips first with a pencil or brush and then filling in the colour. Blot well with a tissue and add some shine with a slick of lip gloss.

10 For a real party face, you could also add some glitter, either to your skin or hair.

Also, don't forget the finishing touch – a good dab or squirt of your favourite scent to make you feel on top of the world!

Cleanse your skin each morning and evening and moisturize generously to prevent your skin drying out. Remember to moisturize your abdomen, too, as this area may become very dry and itchy as the skin is stretched taut.

DIET 8
Frozen food now for healthy meals later

Cook ahead with your freezer
If you have some spare time now, it is a good idea to spend it cooking some dishes ahead to be frozen until after your baby is born. A newborn baby has a fairly intensive routine which does not leave you much time for meal preparation and cooking. A supply of frozen healthy meals ready for defrosting and reheating either in your conventional cooker or microwave oven will be an enormous help. Even after the birth you will have to continue eating really nutritious meals to regain your strength, especially if you are breastfeeding. The milk you supply to your baby is only as good as your diet and the nutrients you get from your everyday food. If you feel tired and harrassed, cooking fresh meals can be a chore and you may be inclined to go without, or eat a convenience snack that is low in nutrients.

Frozen meals can be economical if you use ingredients that are cheap and plentiful in season, especially fruit and vegetables. Most soups, casseroles, pies, quiches, crumbles and even some pasta dishes freeze successfully. Make them up in larger batches than usual, allow to cool thoroughly, then wrap, seal and label.

Frozen food containers
There is a wide range of containers and material that you can use, and your choice will be governed partly by the type of food to be frozen. You need not buy special containers – you can recycle washed-out yoghurt pots, ice-cream tubs and foil containers. However, it is useful to have some of the following:
Foil containers are great for pies and stews and speed up freezing and thawing times.
Plastic containers such as Tupperware are useful for freezing all kinds of food, especially stews, casseroles and soups. Good-quality containers will literally last for ever and never need replacing so they are worth the initial investment.
Freezer bags are usually made of polythene and sold in economical rolls in supermarket and freeze centres. They are ideal for cakes, tarts, pies, bread and other solid items. You can freeze liquid meals in them, too, but it is rather a messy business.
Aluminium foil can be used to wrap pies, tarts, cakes, bread, pastries and other foods to avoid freezer burn, which damages texture and flavour.
Note: all frozen foods should be labelled clearly with the name of the dish and the date frozen for future reference. There is nothing more irritating than hunting through your freezer for a particular item only to be faced with several idential brown-looking frozen blocks of food that you cannot identify. The 'stew' you take out and defrost might well turn out to be soup! Labels will also indicate when certain foods need defrosting and eating before they pass the date of no return.

Freezing rules
1 Never freeze any food until it is completely cold.
2 Always make sure that food is totally wrapped or sealed to prevent freezer burn.
3 Exclude any air if possible from the polythene bag or container for the best results.
4 Always freeze fruit and vegetables when they are really fresh and unbruised. Remember that many need blanching or cooking *before* freezing.
5 Eat food as soon as possible after removing it from the freezer – do not leave it sitting around in the kitchen.
6 The same rule applies to food to be frozen. It should be frozen as soon as it is cool.
7 Defrost food in the refrigerator or a cool place.
8 Never refreeze thawed meat, fish and poultry dishes. If you do not use them soon after defrosting, throw them away.
9 Freeze foods initially in the coldest part of the freezer and then transfer them to another shelf. Only leave the freezer on 'frost-freeze' for 24 hours.
10 Remember when freezing foods to under-season, especially with garlic, as freezing tends to accentuate the natural flavours. Season to taste on reheating.

Foods to avoid
The following do not freeze well:
1 Salad vegetables go soggy and wilted. They are best made into fresh-tasting summer soups and then frozen.
2 Custards tend to separate out.
3 Soufflés, moulds and mousses that contain a lot of gelatine are not very successful.
4 Mayonnaise tends to curdle.
5 Eggs in their shells crack, although the whites and yolks can be frozen separately.

Gazpacho

450g/1lb ripe tomatoes
1 onion, peeled and chopped
1 green pepper, seeded and diced
½ cucumber, chopped
2½ tablespoons stale white breadcrumbs
2 cloves garlic, crushed
2½ tablespoons red wine vinegar
550ml/1 pint tomato juice

Accompaniments:
½ cucumber diced
10 spring onions, chopped
225g/½lb tomatoes, skinned seeded and chopped
1 large green pepper, seeded and chopped

Cut a small cross in the top of the ripe tomatoes, and plunge into boiling water for a few seconds. Carefully peel the skin away from the blanched tomatoes. Discard the skin and roughly chop the tomatoes, removing the tough stalk as you do. Put the roughly chopped tomatoes into a liquidizer or food processor, along with the onion, pepper and cucumber. Blend until finely chopped. Put the chopped vegetables into a bowl with the breadcrumbs, garlic, vinegar and tomato juice. Mix well to blend evenly and allow to stand for 15 minutes. Season the tomato soup well then push through a fine mesh sieve using the back of a wooden spoon and working well to press all the vegetables through, but keeping the pips out of the resulting purée. Chill the soup well before serving with the accompaniments.

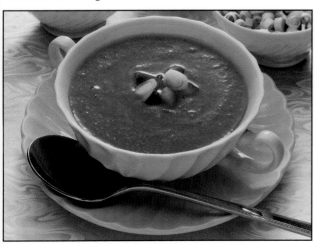

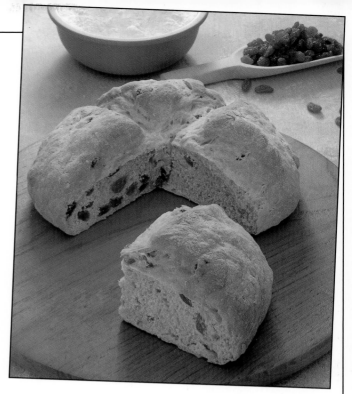

Breads, such as Sultana soda bread (above) and soups, like Gazpacho (below), are tasty and easy to prepare and can be frozen for later when you have less time or energy for cooking.

Sultana soda bread

450g/1lb plain white flour
1¼ teaspoons salt
1¼ teaspoons baking soda
1¼ teaspoons cream of tartar
300ml/½ pint sour milk
100g/4oz sultanas

Sift together the flour, salt, baking soda, and cream of tartar in a mixing bowl. Add the sultanas and mix into the flour quickly, making a slight well in the centre of the flour as you do so. Pour the milk into the well in the flour and mix with a round bladed knife to form a firm but not too stiff dough. Turn the dough onto a lightly floured board and knead quickly. Shape the dough into a ball, and flatten it slightly with the palm of your hand. Place the dough on a lightly greased and floured baking sheet and cut a deep cross into the top of the dough. Bake in a preheated oven at 200°C/400°F/Gas Mark 6 for 25 minutes. After this time, turn the loaf upside down on the baking sheet and return to the oven for a further 10 minutes. Wrap the baked loaf in a damp cloth and place on a wire rack to cool completely.

Frozen food now for healthy meals later

Green pepper soup

3 green peppers, deseeded and chopped
1 large onion, chopped
15g/¹/₂oz/1 tablespoon margarine
550ml/1 pint/2¹/₂ cups vegetable stock
salt and pepper
good pinch basil or oregano
300ml/¹/₂ pint/1¹/₄ cups white sauce
chopped parsley and croûtons to garnish

Sauté the pepper and onion in the fat until soft. Add the stock, seasoning and herbs and simmer for 15-20 minutes. Liquidize and return to the pan. Stir the sauce into the soup and heat gently. Cool and freeze when completely cold. To serve, defrost and reheat. Serve sprinkled with parsley and croûtons. Serves 4.

Cornish pasties

450g/1lb/4¹/₂ cups self-raising wholemeal flour
100g/4oz/¹/₂ cup mixed lard and margarine
60ml/4 tablespoons water
beaten egg for glazing
Filling:
2 large potatoes
1 medium swede
350g/12oz chuck steak or skirt, diced
2 onions, chopped
salt and freshly ground black pepper
small knob of lard

Make the pastry in the usual way. Knead lightly and put aside to rest. Peel the potatoes and swede and grate coarsely with the cucumber grating side of the grater, or peel into strips with a potato peeler.

Roll out the pastry and cut into 4 ovals. Place the rolling pin half-way under an oval and droop the pastry on either side. Using the rolling pin as a divider and back-rest, start piling up the filling on one side, starting with the potato, then the swede, steak and lastly the onion. Sprinkle with lots of freshly ground pepper and salt and place tiny knobs of lard along the top. This will keep the pastry moist during cooking. Dampen the edges of the pastry and fold the top over to meet the bottom. Seal the edges securely, pressing between finger and thumb. Curl the edges back and 'plait' them so that they are sealed and no filling or meat juices can leak out during cooking. Place on a well-greased baking sheet and brush with beaten egg. Assemble the other pasties. Bake in a preheated oven at 180°C, 350°F, gas 4 for 1³/₄-2 hours until the pastry is golden and cooked. Leave to cool. Wrap in foil and freeze. To reheat, defrost, then place the pasties on a baking sheet, cover with foil and heat in a medium oven.

Pork steaks in orange sauce

300ml/2 tablespoons oil
2 onions, thinly sliced
15g/¹/₂oz/1 tablespoon butter
5ml/1 teaspoon Dijon mustard
15ml/1 tablespoon soft brown sugar
grated rind of 2 oranges
4 pork steaks
30ml/2 tablespoons flour
300ml/¹/₂ pint/1¹/₄ cups chicken stock
150ml/¹/₄ pint/⁵/₈ cup white wine or cider
juice of 2 oranges
salt and pepper
100g/4oz button mushrooms, sliced
1 large orange, peeled and segmented

Heat the oil in a flameproof casserole dish and sauté the onion until soft. Remove from the pan and keep warm. Mix the butter, mustard, sugar and orange rind to a thick paste. Add to the pan with the pork steaks and sauté until browned on both sides. Remove and keep warm. Stir the flour into the pan juices and cook for 3 minutes. Add the stock and wine, a little at a time, stirring until the sauce thickens. Bring to the boil, add the orange juice and seasoning and return the onions and meat to the pan. Cover and place in a preheated oven at 180°C, 350°F, gas 4 for about 1¹/₄-1¹/₂ hours. Add the mushrooms to the casserole about 10 minutes before the end of cooking time. Add the orange segments. Cool and freeze. Defrost and heat in a medium oven. Serves 4.

Moussaka with yoghurt

2 large aubergines/eggplants, thinly sliced
olive oil for frying

2 onions, chopped
30ml/2 tablespoons oil
450g/1lb minced lean lamb
450g/1lb canned tomatoes
5ml/1 teaspoon brown sugar
15ml/1 tablespoon oregano
2.5ml/½ teaspoon each of ground cinnamon,
allspice and cumin
50g/2oz/¾ cup dried apricots, soaked overnight
30ml/2 tablespoons tomato paste
60ml/4 tablespoons pine nuts
50ml/2floz/¼ cup red wine or stock
100g/4oz feta cheese, crumbled
30ml/2 tablespoons grated Parmesan cheese
Yoghurt topping:
150ml/¼ pint/⅝ cup natural yoghurt
2 eggs, beaten
50ml/2floz/¼ cup milk

Spread the sliced aubergine/eggplant out in a colander and sprinkle with salt. Leave for 30 minutes to exude any excess moisture. Rinse in cold water and pat dry. Fry gently in a little olive oil until golden-brown. Drain and set aside. Make the meat sauce: sauté the onion in the oil until soft. Add the lamb and brown it. Add the tomatoes and their juice, sugar, herbs, spices, chopped apricots and tomato paste. Bring to the boil and cook rapidly for about 15 minutes until the sauce thickens. Stir in the pine nuts and red wine. Season to taste. Grease a shallow ovenproof dish and arrange in it layers of aubergine and meat sauce. Crumble the feta cheese across the top. Beat the yoghurt, eggs and milk together and season. Pour over the moussaka and sprinkle with Parmesan cheese. Bake uncovered in a preheated oven at 180°C, 350°F, gas 4 for 45-50 minutes, until the topping is set, golden-brown and slightly risen. Leave to cool, cover with foil and freeze. Defrost and reheat in a moderate oven. Serve with a green salad.

Wholemeal fatless sponge cake

75g/3oz/⅜ cup soft brown sugar
3 large eggs
75g/3oz/¾ cup wholemeal flour
jam and cream for filling
caster sugar for dusting

Whisk the sugar and eggs until they leave a 'trail' from the beaters of the whisk. Fold in the flour, a little at a time, with a metal spoon. Do not over-mix. Butter two 17.5cm/7in sandwich cake tins and line the bases with greaseproof paper. Pour in the sponge mixture, smooth the top and bake in a preheated oven at 190°C, 375°F, gas 5 on the middle shelf for about 25 minutes until well-risen and cooked. Allow to cool on a wire cake rack. Sandwich the sponges together with your favourite filling and dust the top with sugar.

Date slices

100g/4oz/1¼ cups wholemeal flour
5ml/1 teaspoon bicarbonate of soda
150/5oz/⅝ cup margarine
25g/1oz/⅓ cup wheatgerm
25g/1oz/⅓ cup dessicated coconut
25g/1oz/¼ cup chopped nuts
75g/3oz/⅜ cup molasses sugar
100g/4oz/1⅓ cups oats
150g/5oz/1 cup chopped dried dates
15ml/1 tablespoon dark rum
30ml/2 tablespoons honey

Mix the flour, a pinch of salt and bicarbonate of soda and rub in the margarine. Stir in the wheatgerm, coconut, nuts, molasses sugar and oats. Press half of the mixture into a 19cm/7½in square shallow, greased baking tin. Press down firmly.

Simmer the dates gently with the rum and honey for a few minutes. Spread the date mixture over the crumble mixture and cover with the rest of the crumble, pressing down firmly. Bake in a preheated oven at 180°C, 350°F, gas 4 for 30 minutes. Cut into slices and cool in the tin. Makes 10 slices.

Banana bread

75g/3oz/⅜ cup margarine
150g/5oz/⅝ cup soft brown sugar
2 large ripe bananas, mashed
150ml/¼ pint/⅝ cup natural yoghurt
1 egg, beaten
200g/7oz/2 cups wholemeal flour
7.5ml/1½ teaspoons bicarbonate of soda
15ml/1 tablespoon chopped nuts

Cream the fat and sugar, then gradually mix in the banana, yoghurt and beaten egg. Fold in the flour, a pinch of salt and bicarbonate of soda. Beat well. Spoon into a well-greased baking tin and scatter the nuts over the top. Bake in a preheated oven at 180°C, 350°F, gas 4 for about 1 hour. Allow to cool and serve sliced and buttered. Makes 1 loaf.

Practise your breathing for labour

This month's exercise section focuses on breathing exercises. These are potentially the most important exercises you can perform during pregnancy if you are planning a natural birth without recourse to pain-killing drugs. Breathing will help carry you through labour and enable you to cope with pain. You have probably practised some of these exercises at antenatal classes. If you haven't, it is never too late to start and you should make them part of your daily ritual from now on until the big day arrives and your baby is born.

Before you start, put on something comfortable – a leotard and tights, a loose tracksuit or baggy dungarees. Sit cross-legged or in the tailor sitting position (shown in the pictures) on the floor in a warm room. You will find that this is one of the easiest and most comfortable ways to sit during pregnancy. It rounds out and eases your spine and it helps boost blood circulation in your legs and feet. It also stretches out the inner thigh muscles and loosens your groin, both of which are beneficial in labour itself.

You will find that this position is very relaxing and aids good breathing. However, if you find it difficult to hold for any length of time and get uncomfortable, you can lie back with your head, shoulders and upper back supported by some cushions or pillows and practise the breathing exercises in exactly the same way.

It is well known that the way in which you breathe is related to your emotional state and the degree of pain you are feeling. Thus if you are tense, upset, angry or in pain, you will probably breathe more quickly in shorter, shallower breaths and take in less air. When you are happy, content and relaxed, you tend to breathe more slowly and deeply. During labour you need to make your breathing work for you and not against you in a positive way. Establishing regulated, steady rhythms which are practised over and over again until they become automatic and almost second nature, will stand you in good stead. They will enable you to relax between contractions and to cope with the pain during a labour contraction. Staying calm and relaxed will

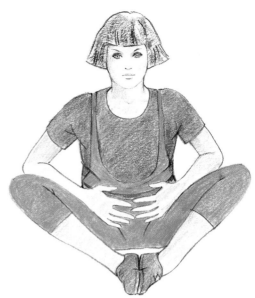

1 *Practise your breathing exercises in the tailor sitting position. Sit on a flat surface with back straight and the soles of your feet pressed together. This is easier than it looks. Place both hands on your abdomen and breathe in slowly through your nose. Exhale through your nose or mouth, trying to relax your abdominal muscles as you breathe out.*

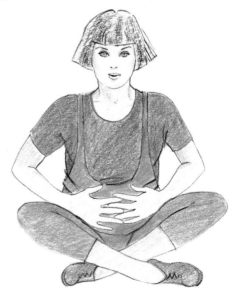

2 *Try practising this abdominal breathing sitting in a more conventional cross-legged position. Press lightly on your sides to feel how the muscles respond during breathing.*

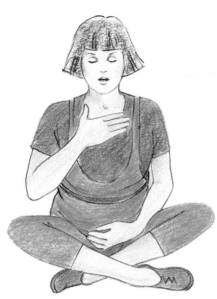

3 Practise panting to help you deal with the peak of a contraction. Quicker breathing and shallower breaths will help surmount the pain. Gradually slow this down into more rhythmic breathing as the contraction subsides. Try inhaling quickly 2-3 times, sigh, then pant. Place your hand on your upper chest as you pant and feel it moving.

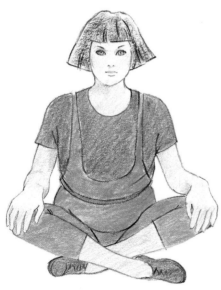

4 Practise breathing through a contraction in a cross-legged position with your hands resting on your knees. Relax your abdominal muscles as your chest rises and falls.

help you to overcome tension and fear and also enable you to preserve your strength during labour for the real work of expulsion (when the baby is born and you push her out). It is easy to get worn out in the first stage of labour so that you are ill-prepared for the effort required in the second stage.

You will find that as labour progresses and the contractions get closer together that you will automatically breathe more quickly and deeply. This may cause you to hyperventilate and can lead to dizziness or a black-out as carbon-dioxide leaves your bloodstream.

Breathing and relaxation cannot be separated, and for conscious relaxation routines and exercises, turn to page 144. In labour, you will need to breathe according to the degree of relaxation or pain you feel. It is essential that you should always be in control of your body and what is happening, and the way to do this is by controlling your breathing. Practice over the next few weeks will help you build up confidence so that you fear the prospect of labour less and can actually welcome it, because you have practised and rehearsed what is to come and know that you *can* cope.

Some women panic when the contractions become more powerful and come faster, and succumb totally to the pain and emotion of the moment. There is no need to feel ashamed of this – women can experience different levels of pain and react accordingly, and if you want to seek pain relief to escape these powerful, compelling waves then there is no point prolonging the 'suffering' unnecessarily. However, if you accept what is happening and make up your mind that you are not going to fight the natural forces within your body but are going to ride them out and control them, then you will need to know the following breathing techniques. Do not be fooled into thinking that they have magic properties and will dispel the pain completely. They just enable you to cope with labour more effectively and less fearfully and to experience it more fully.

The exercises
You will find it helpful if you are aware of the way in which your muscles work during breathing. Rest your hands on your chest, diaphragm and abdomen as indicated in the drawings to increase this awareness. As you breathe, look down at your body and study the way your chest rises and falls. As you inhale (breathe in) your body noticeably expands. As you exhale (breathe out), it contracts. Practise

Practise your breathing for labour

inhaling deeply, slowly and rhythmically with one hand resting on your upper chest, the other on your abdomen. Try inhaling through your nose and exhaling through your mouth in a long, slow release of air. Control your breathing all the time.

Now you are ready to start the exercises themselves that you will use during labour. When you feel a contraction beginning, you will start breathing out slowly. Then breathe slowly and rhythmically through the contraction – it lasts about 45 seconds to one minute. As it slowly starts to fade away, you can breathe out slowly through your mouth and then relax and rest.

As the contractions get stronger and more frequent at the end of the first stage of labour, you will need to pant, too. Imagine that the contraction is starting and breathe rhythmically as before. As the contraction builds up change to panting in faster, shallower breaths. If you place your hand on the upper part of your chest you will feel it moving gently. Pant about once every second to get you through the strongest part of the contraction and then relax into the rhythmic breathing again, finishing with a final long, slow exhalation of air through your mouth. Relax.

It may help when you practise these exercises if you imagine that the contractions are like waves which you are jumping over in the sea. The wave gradually builds up until it is high and crashes over you (when you need to pant at the height of a contraction) and then it gradually subsides and slowly ebbs away. Do not allow the wave to carry you away – ride it instead and stay in control. Practise this 'peaks and troughs' breathing with your partner. He can help coach you through your labour and encourage you when the pain is great and you are on the point of giving into it and flowing with it rather than riding it.

Relaxing the abdominal muscles during labour
Incorrect breathing can cause your abdominal muscles to contract and become tense during a contraction which will make you feel more uncomfortable. Therefore, it is helpful to know how

to relax these muscles. Lie back on some cushions and place both hands on your lower abdomen. As you breathe out slowly and then in, feel your abdomen and chest expanding. Try to relax your abdominal muscles as you breathe out. Really concentrate hard on getting this right. As your abdomen becomes more relaxed and moves less, your breathing will get progressively faster and not so deep and you will feel less abdominal discomfort.

You can go one stage further and practise slow chest breathing instead. This is more suitable for the end of the first stage of labour when you are almost fully dilated and will soon be ready to push the baby out. This type of breathing takes the strain off your abdomen and utilises the muscles higher up between the ribs in your chest. Place both hands on your rib cage with your fingertips just touching. As you breathe in and your ribs expand, your fingertips will separate. As you breathe out and your chest relaxes, your fingertips will touch. Consciously try to breathe with the muscles of your chest only so that your abdomen moves less.

Working with your partner
As described above, it can be extremely reassuring and comforting to be 'coached' through labour by your partner, and it is a good idea to practise the exercises together. One way to build up a working relationship and closeness for labour is through touch relaxation. This term applies to the ways in which you can relax by responding to your partner's touch. Gentle stroking and massage of your arms, back and shoulders in particular can be very soothing and relaxing. It also enables your partner to sense whether you are tense or relaxed and to help you through your labour accordingly.

Sit propped up against some cushions and ask your partner to start stroking your arm with both hands from your shoulder to your hand, gently increasing the pressure as he builds up the strokes. Try to relax and flow with the direction of your partner's hands. Do not tighten your muscles or resist his stroking. In this way he can gradually work round your body – your arms, shoulders, back, abdomen and legs.

Practise this routine regularly – it is enjoyable for both of you and gradually you will get accustomed to relaxing when your partner strokes you. It builds up co-operation between you so that when the big day comes you can really work together as a team. Your partner will have the pleasure of really participating in a positive way in the birth process

1 This shows breathing during the gentle contractions at the start of labour, before you leave for hospital. Breathe rhythmically – not too deep or fast – and try to relax into the contractions. Stand, lie down or bend over, whichever you find most comfortable.

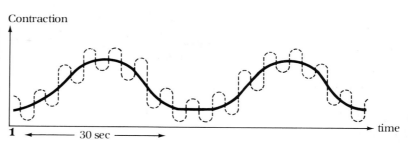

2 Increase rate of breathing as contractions become stronger. Breathe faster and shallower in the upper part of your chest at the peak of the contraction when relaxation becomes harder. At this stage you may find sitting down more comfortable.

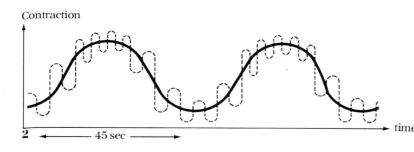

3 At the end of the first stage of your labour the contractions become longer and more intense. Breathe in groups of three: in-out, in-out, in-sigh. It may help to lie on your side and you may want to push. Panting may help if you are not yet fully dilated.

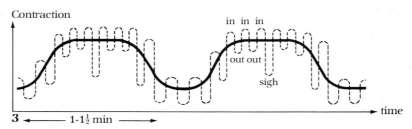

and knowing that he can be a comfort and source of strength to you, and it will be reassuring for you to have him present and helping. He can help you relax, coach you through the contractions, steady your breathing and encourage you to keep on going. If you can respond to his touch and trust in him, there will be no need for spoken words and instructions.

Some practical points about massage

You need not take your clothes off although it is often more effective on bare skin. You will react faster to skin-to-skin contact. It is easier to use an aromatherapy oil, moisturizing lotion or even talcum powder rather than stroking bare skin. A moisturizer is particularly soothing and will give you a luxurious beauty treatment at the same time, especially on any areas of dry or flaky skin such as your abdomen. As this gets larger and the skin stretches, it can become very dry and itchy and fall prey to stretch marks.

It goes without saying that you should do this in a warm room and make yourself comfortable first. Prop yourself up with cushions, sit cross-legged or lie on your side – whatever position is most relaxing. Do not rush and treat it as a chore – think of it rather as a time for relaxing together.

Learn the art of conscious relaxation

As your pregnancy progresses and your abdomen swells, you will need to spend more time each day relaxing. This can be a stressful time for many women and it is important to build a quiet period into your usual daily routine specifically for relaxation. This does not mean just lying down on a sofa in front of the television with your feet up – although this may give your legs a rest, it is not necessary relaxing. Real relaxation is a fusion of both

body and mind. It is a conscious exercise like yoga, meditation or slow, full breathing. Of course, curling up in bed with a good book or wallowing in a warm bath are relaxing but they are not necessarily calming. They may relax your body but they cannot reduce the stresses of a busy day at work, say, that exist in your mind. They are only a temporary respite.

If you used to smoke or drink to help induce a calm, relaxed state of mind, you may have special problems relaxing now if you gave up these habits when you discovered that you were pregnant. You, in particular, need to find alternative positive ways to relax. If you are still working full-time or have personal or financial problems of any kind, you may be under considerable stress and be very tense. Learning the relaxation skills outlined here will be exceptionally valuable to you and may help you to see all your problems in a new light and to find ways of surmounting them.

If you are the sort of person who likes to be busy all the time doing things and enjoying a lot of activity, then it may be very difficult for you to understand that quiet periods of relaxation can be beneficial and worthwhile. You have to believe that you are not wasting time when you relax. On the contrary, you are giving your body a real pick-me-up,

Yoga is an excellent way of relaxing as it is a conscious exercise that involves the interaction of both your mind and your body. It can help keep you calm and prepare you for childbirth by teaching you good breathing and how to relax between contractions. Sit cross-legged as here, or try the classic lotus position. Yoga might be a good alternative for relaxation if, before pregnancy, you were used to smoking or drinking alcohol to help keep you calm.

and for after the birth too when your baby may be very demanding, and you will feel drained and exhausted and need to snatch short periods of total relaxation in order to recover.

The most important reason, however, for learning how to relax is the way in which it can help you during the delivery of your baby in a really positive way. Relaxation and correct breathing go hand in hand. You will need to try and stay calm and in control of your body when the contractions start, and especially so when they build up into the second stage of labour. Practising the art of gentle relaxation now will help you to stay calm under the physical and mental pressures of childbirth and cope better with any pain you may experience.

Calm, laid-back mothers tend to have more easy tempered babies as a rule. It seems that most babies

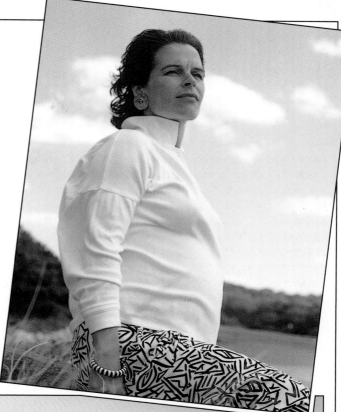

At this stage of your pregnancy you should spend some time relaxing every day. Whenever you get the opportunity try to stop and rest, or lie down and put your feet up. Elevating your legs will boost circulation and prevent pooling of blood in the lower legs, thus helping to prevent varicose veins.

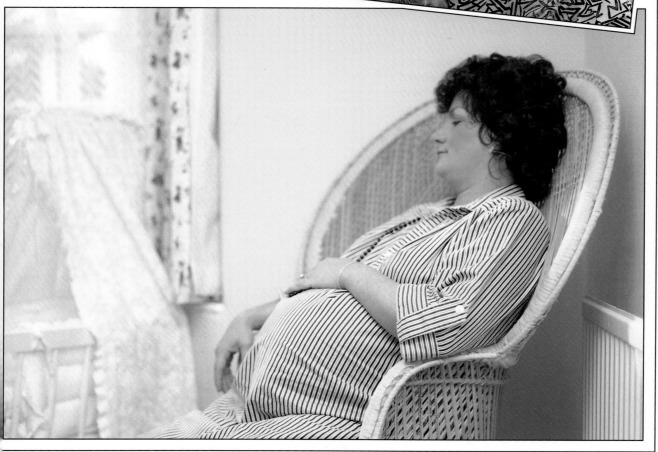

Learn the art of conscious relaxation

thrive and are more content when their mothers are naturally calm and relaxed, both during pregnancy and after delivery. These mothers seem to transmit their essential inner tranquility to their children. There is no doubt that babies are very receptive to their mothers' moods, so here is another reason for practising conscious relaxation. If you are feeling tired and harassed with the constant demands of coping with a newborn baby, you can put her down to sleep and rejuvenate yourself by stealing a few minutes of deep, total relaxation to set you up before the next round of feeds and changes.

Relaxation does not necessarily come naturally – it requires concentration, dedication and practice. If you have not already started by now, the eighth month of pregnancy, you should not delay any more. You may have been taught some basics already if you are attending antenatal classes. Remember that relaxation should combine your body and mind. It is important to cut out all external noises and distractions and focus solely on your inner self. This in itself is a useful exercise for labour when you may wish to shut out the sounds of other women giving birth nearby.

Most relaxation exercises involve lying down on the floor or a bed, so you should make sure that you will be comfortable and warm. You may need some pillows or cushions to support your head and shoulders, knees or abdomen. The room should be warm or you should be dressed warmly in loose, comfortable clothing. If necessary, take off your watch or remove the clock from the room so that you are not tempted to count the minutes and thus hinder relaxation. When you take up any of the positions mentioned here, you should try to relax and let your limbs go loose. Do not tense any muscles.

Toe to top exercise
Lie on your side on the floor with your head and shoulders supported by cushions and another one placed strategically under a knee. This is a better position for relaxation than lying on your back especially in the later months of pregnancy when

your uterus may press on the main blood vessels in a lying flat position. Now you are going to consciously and gradually relax your whole body, starting at your feet and working upwards along your legs and torso to your head until you are totally relaxed. Focus on your toes, move them about a little and flex and relax them. Now work upwards stretching and relaxing your ankle, legs, hips and pelvis, your abdomen, chest, arms, shoulders and finally your facial muscles so that your whole body is free from tension. All the while, think of yourself and your baby, and her closeness to you. When you feel really relaxed, try to wipe your mind free of conflicting thoughts and emotions. Either concentrate on making it go completely blank or you can try focusing on a single object or thought to the exclusion of all others. Stay like this for about 10 minutes or so and then start regaining control of your body upwards from your feet to your head. Now stretch out as far as you can go and relax.

Another way of performing this relaxation exercise is to start in the centre of your body at your pelvis. Press it down into the floor and relax it. Now work downwards, pressing and relaxing your muscles alternately, and then upwards from the pelvis to your face on the same principle. Try to make your body feel really limp and floppy and let go.

Breathing relaxation
Focusing on your breathing is another way of relaxing and one that will stand you in good stead for labour. The way in which you breathe can help clear your consciousness, eliminating tensions from your mind and body and making you feel more calm and restful. Breathing is the key to changing your energy level and your mood in both yoga and meditation. You may have noticed how when you are tense you tend to breathe quickly in small shallow gasps. Breathing in this way does not allow sufficient oxygen to be absorbed into the bloodstream, and thus the amount available for meeting the needs of your heart and other organs, nerves, brain and skin and those of your baby is restricted. Your body is not working efficiently and you may feel tired and dispirited.

But the opposite is true when you relax – you tend to breathe more slowly and deeply. You inhale more oxygen to supply your body's needs and thus you feel calmer, more comfortable and your vitality increases. You have more energy thanks to higher levels of oxygen in your bloodstream, cells and tissues. If you don't believe it, just try it out when you next feel angry, upset or tense – deliberately breathe more slowly, taking in deep lungfuls of air and breathing with your whole chest and abdomen. As you inhale more oxygen, you will start to feel calmer.

Most of the world's great religions and philosophies have attached special importance to breathing, and it is associated traditionally with power and energy. Thus in the Bible the Holy Spirit is the breath of God. The Latin word for breath is *spiritus*, and the definition of spirit is the life force that animates the bodies of all living things. There can be no life without breath. In yoga, breathing is harnessed to meditation to control the mind and the body and even to overcome pain itself.

In childbirth, breathing will not guarantee total relaxation nor relief from pain but it certainly can help you to cope with the discomfort and pain and to be in control of your body and mind. If you can automatically associate relaxation with the way in which you breathe, you will be able to relax more deeply between contractions when you need to recover and rest, and conserve your energy for stage two when the baby is born.

Regular breathing exercises can also help you to develop greater lung capacity. You may find that you start to feel generally more relaxed and healthy within yourself with increased energy. There could even be beauty spin-offs as your hair and skin can benefit from more oxygen flowing to the cells and a more efficient removal of wastes from your system. When you are lying down in the exercise described earlier (toe to head) try to focus on your breathing. Really concentrate on the air you are inhaling, breathing in slowly through your nose and then exhaling equally slowly through your mouth in a long drawn-out sigh. The reason for this is that breathing air in through your mouth during labour may make your throat very dry. Be aware of the way in which your chest gently rises and falls and listen to the natural rhythm of your breathing.

Yoga

I have mentioned yoga before in this book but it has a special significance in the art of relaxation as it seeks to establish a total union or integration of mind, body and spirit. It is an extension of meditation in that it promotes enlightenment through exercising and training the body as well as the mind. According to yoga theory we all have two different kinds of energy – male energy which is stimulating, dynamic and creative; and female energy which is restoring, gentle and calming. These two energies are imbalanced in most people, but yoga strives to release both and bring them into harmony and balance. This is reflected in the yoga postures, or *asanas*. Most of the exercises that are performed standing up are strengthening and relate to male energy, whereas the gentler, more relaxing seated or lying down asanas are more female oriented.

Yoga tries to remove tension, release energy and encourage and foster creativity. It reduces stress, helps you to sleep better and leaves you feeling calm and relaxed. You can then channel this energy into other areas of your life. Breathing plays an important role as it is the link between body and mind. It can help relax your muscles as well as relieving mental tension and stress. It aids circulation and blood flow to the brain and muscles and has a tranquilizing effect. So you can see again that yoga could prepare you in a very positive way for the experience of labour. It will also stretch out your muscles, make you more flexible, help develop strength and endurance and make you feel generally more energetic – all the qualities you will need for an easier delivery.

You can try relaxing in the classic yoga lotus position or sitting cross-legged on the floor with your hands resting on your knees. This is surprisingly comfortable, rounds out your back and helps dispel any tension in the spinal area. Or you can adopt the yoga 'corpse' position which is used to strengthen the body. In this form of deep relaxation, your mind and body should be joined together in perfect unity. You can either lie flat on your back on the floor or, better still, on a slanting board with the raised end resting about 30cm/12in above ground level. Lie with your head at the bottom and your feet at the top and slowly relax your body from your toes to your head. Maintain this position for 10-15 minutes and then gradually regain control and relax. It has the other advantage of raising your legs and helping prevent varicose veins. It helps make you feel more energetic and reduces aches and pains in your body. If you don't have a slanting board you can just lie on the floor with your feet resting on a chair or a low table, or even up against the wall itself. Place a cushion strategically in the small of your back to prevent any discomfort. After the period of relaxation you can practise a few buttocks lifts or pelvic floor exercises while you remain in this position.

Shop ahead for a fashionable baby

Your baby's shopping list

If you have not already done so, you should go out and buy some clothes and basic items for your new baby. You may be surprised at how expensive baby things are, but it is possible to buy them second-hand at a fraction of the cost, and you may have friends or relations who have completed their families and have spare baby clothes and equipment that they can lend or donate.

Although babies are only little people, they need a lot of things, it is best to plan ahead now and buy them before the birth. You may feel very tired next month anyway and won't want to trail around shops buying prams and babygrowers. Be prepared so that when you bring your baby home, everything is ready and waiting and there are no hiccups.

Get the nursery ready

Although you may put the baby down to sleep in your own bedroom for the first two or three weeks to make night feeds easier, you will soon feel the need for your own privacy and some peace and quiet, and will want her to have her own room. A small bedroom can be decorated with pretty paint or children's wallpaper and furnishings in readiness for the new baby. A crib or cradle, preferably one that rocks to encourage sleep, is ideal for the first three months or so but then she will need a larger cot. Make sure that the crib or cot is fitted with a proper safety mattress with air holes and a cover.

You will also need several cot sheet as they frequently get damp! And some cot blankets and a quilt or eiderdown. Babies don't need pillows – they sleep quite happily on their sides or backs. A pillow can be dangerous and may cause them to suffocate. Also, until their spines and necks are stronger (at least one year), it is better for them to sleep absolutely flat. A pretty quilted cot bumper will keep out draughts and stop an older baby crashing her head against the bars. However, some babies find it infuriating if it prevents them seeing out through the

Baby checklist
Here is a useful shopping list for you to refer to and tick off the items you need to buy. You don't have to rush out and buy them all, but many will prove useful and can be stocked up in readiness for your home-coming.

1 Sleeping
crib/cot
sheets (5-6)
blankets (3)
quilt/eiderdown
cot bumper
cot mattress + cover
nightlight
cot mobiles
baby alarm

2 Clothing
stretchsuits (5-6)
vests (5-6)
plastic waterproof pants (5-6)
pyjamas or nighties (4)
socks
bootees
hat or bonnet
mittens
jacket
cardigans (4-5)
romper suit
dress
dungarees
T-shirts/shorts

3 Nappy changing
24 terry towelling nappies
smallest size disposable nappies (3 packs)
nappy safety pins
nappy liners
creams or ointment
wet-wipes for travelling
baby lotion for cleansing
cotton wool balls
nappy bucket with lid
sanitizing powder or fluid
changing mat

4 Travelling
pram
reclining pushchair
pram bedding
baby sling with head support
carry-cot/moses basket
restraint reins for car seat
apron/hood for pushchair
snug travel bag – zipped and quilted
bag for baby's things

5 Feeding
nursing bras (2)
breast pads
feeding bottles + teats
electric bottle warmer
polystyrene travelling bottle container
sterilizer
bottle brush
sterilizing fluid or tablets
formula milk
juice – non-sweetened
baby vitamin drops
gripe water
soft muslin squares to catch drips

6 Amusements
mobiles
pram beads
bouncing cradle
nursery rhyme tapes
womb noise tape

7 Bathing
baby bath + back rest
baby bath foam
towels
flannels
talcum powder
baby oil
baby shampoo

cot bars. If it spoils your baby's view and enrages her, adjust or remove it.

In the nursery, you will also need a changing mat for changing nappies and drying the baby, and a nearby supply of nappies, pins, creams and plastic pants. You can buy a special baby dresser at waist level with pockets and drawers for all these items but it is not essential. The baby's clothes can be stored away neatly in a small chest.

A colourful mobile that turns in the breeze can be hung above the cot to keep the baby amused, and a musical box that plays Brahms' Lullaby or some other soothing tune will help send her to sleep (you hope!). Meanwhile, a nightlight will enable you to see your way round her room in the dark and may be bright enough for changing nappies. Turning on the main electric light is guaranteed to really awaken a sleepy baby. And a baby alarm with a microphone operated by batteries will ensure that you hear your baby if she cries in the night.

Keeping your baby warm and chic

Baby clothes are now very colourful and fashionable – the days of bootees, bonnets and matinée jackets tied with ribbons and bows are fading fast, and even the tiniest babies can be trendily turned out if you wish. Your baby will need a supply of vests with wide neck openings and preferably buttoning under the nappy to prevent any bare midriffs. All-in-one stretchsuits are ideal for newborn babies and keep them warm and snug. Don't fuss about colours – blue, white, pastel greens and red suit boys *and* girls! You can put on little cardigans or jackets over the top in cold weather. Your baby may also need socks, and definitely a soft shawl to wrap her up in. In a hot summer, a tiny baby can live in vests and romper suits or little dresses. Make sure she is neither too hot nor too cold at any time. And outside on a cold day, keep her head covered to prevent chills.

However, underneath the fashionable accessories your baby will still need a nappy, whether its a terry towelling job or a disposable. The choice is your's – most modern mums favour disposable while nannies like the good old terries. Disposable are best when you are in a hurry, haven't a washing machine or are going out somewhere with the baby, but terries are preferable at night as they are more absorbent and softer to wear. If you use terries, be sure to soak them in sterilizing solution before washing and use a

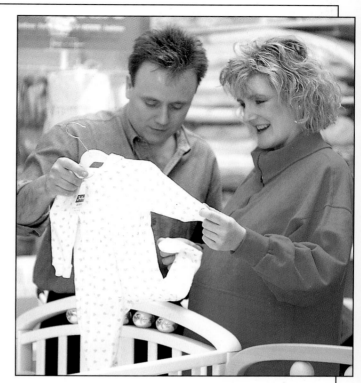

It can be fun shopping for baby clothes. They come in a wide range of colours, fabrics and designs. Alternatively you can experiment with knitting or sewing different outfits yourself.

non-biological washing powder which will not irritate your baby's ultra-sensitive skin. You will also need a nappy pail and some liners.

Travelling with your baby

The most traditional way of travelling with a baby is a pram. Large bouncy ones rarely fold down to be stored away in cars, so you may find that a carry-cot top on a buggy base or a fully reclining pushchair is most handy. You will need bedding for the pram, too, and your baby can sleep in it in the house or garden during the day. If you use a fully reclining buggy, make sure that it has a plastic hood and apron for protection against rain and cold winds.

Even small babies can be carried in a sling against your chest. Many prefer this means of transport as they feel warm and comfortable snuggled up against you, and the more upright position helps bring up any wind and prevent stomach aches. When carrying your baby in the car put the carry-cot on the back seat and support it with a special safety restraint strap to keep it rigid.

The months of waiting are over

You

The last month and you probably cannot wait to be free of your 'bump' and meet your baby in the flesh. The baby moves less in the last few weeks and you may find that you only receive the odd kick now. Meanwhile, your cervix is getting ready for labour and the Braxton-Hicks contractions will be getting stronger and a little more uncomfortable. Now is the time to give up work if you have not already done so and take it easy – make sure that you get adequate rest and sleep every day leading up to the birth. You need it now for your sake *and* that of the baby – and it may cause problems if you suddenly go into labour in the middle of a meeting at the office or on a crowded commuter bus or train!

Many women worry about labour now – especially first-time mothers. Will it be unbearably painful? Will I be able to cope? How will I recognize the onset of labour? The antenatal classes should have helped to prepare you for what is to come, and the breathing exercises and relaxation techniques you have practised will stand you in good stead. Everybody experiences some degree of discomfort or pain, but the more relaxed you feel and the healthier and fitter you are, the easier your labour will be. Needless worry and apprehension will only make things worse than they really are.

Nor should you worry that labour will start without you realizing it. You will know that the time has come to leave for hospital when you experience one of the following:

1 Your waters break – the membranes rupture and release fluid. If this happens you should leave for the hospital right away as the baby is less well protected and more vulnerable to infection.

2 You may have a 'show' – you lose the bloodstained mucus plug from the neck of the womb. This is often the forerunner of labour and may be accompanied by low backache.

3 You may experience regular contractions of increasing length and frequency. And when they come about once every five minutes and last for over 40 seconds you should leave immediately for the hospital – even earlier if you have a long journey.

These illustrations show the progress of the baby through the birth canal into the world outside.

1 The cervix is almost completely dilated here towards the end of the first stage of labour although the bag of water is still intact. By the time the cervix has dilated to 9-10cm, you will get the urge to bear down and push your baby out.

2 In the second stage of labour you have to work hard to push your baby out. Eventually her head will appear in the birth opening with the face turned towards your back.

3 The baby's head emerges, and she slides out through the perineum as you push out the shoulders. It is a marvellous sensation to feel your child being born and to hold her in your arms at last.

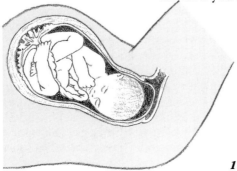

1

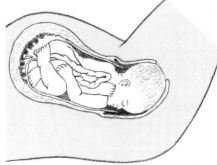

2

Do not forget to take your bag with you, which should be packed and ready. You will want to change and freshen up after the baby is born.

Most women find it a great comfort and help to have their partners with them at this time, giving them encouragement and being generally loving and reassuring. They can help, too, by massaging an aching back or actively coaching you through your labour. Although many men feel slightly squeamish or awkward about being present at the birth of their babies, most find the experience enormously rewarding and would not miss it for the world. You cannot insist that your man is present but do tell him how much it would mean to you and how you would appreciate his presence. Most hospitals now encourage fathers to attend the delivery and even to assist actively in the birth in some cases!

When it is all over, you can hold your baby for a short time before a well-earned rest. Now you can look forward to getting to know your baby, feeding her and caring for her, and getting back to normal.

Your baby

The average baby weighs about 3.4kg/7lb at birth and may be born any time between the thirty-eighth and forty-second weeks. As the birth draws nearer, the baby settles down lower in your pelvis and engages ready for the big moment. She also practises her breathing movements and, as amniotic fluid passes into her trachea, she may have hiccups. She is now ready to start her journey through the birth canal into the outside world.

During the first stage of labour the uterine contractions help the cervix dilate and open around the baby's head. When it is fully dilated (about 10cm) the second stage of labour can commence and the baby's head passes into the top of the vagina. When this happens you will feel a strong urge to bear down and push the baby out. Eventually, her head will 'crown' – appear through the vaginal opening – and then a few seconds later the shoulders and the rest of the body will slide out.

Do not be alarmed if the baby appears slightly bluish in colour, or her head is a strange shape due to an awkward passage into the world. These things will soon rectify themselves. As she breathes normally, she will turn pink. Just hold her and enjoy her – this is an important part of the bonding process between mother and child.

In the third and final stage of labour, the placenta – the baby's life-support system during pregnancy – is delivered and then it is all over. At last you can relax and enjoy being a mother.

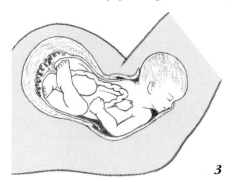

3

Get your bag packed

Make sure that during this month your overnight bag is packed ready to leave in a hurry if need be. Include the following:

1 Front-opening nightdresses
2 Dressing gown or housecoat
3 Front-fastening bras
4 Breastpads
5 Salt
6 Maternity pads
7 Disposable pants
8 Washbag and make-up
9 Towels
10 Slippers

Massage away aches and pains and tension

The months of waiting are nearly over and the baby is due any week now. You probably can hardly wait for the big day to arrive when you finally hold her in your arms. To avoid boredom and take your mind off any discomfort you may be feeling it is important to keep busy. If you are still working full-time, now may be the time to pack it in and to enjoy a few days or weeks relaxation. During this last month the womb lowers and the baby's head engages in the pelvis, and you will probably feel a little more comfortable. Any breathlessness will become a thing of the past.

Massage away backache

Backache may be a problem now and also later on in labour. Pay attention to your posture when sitting and standing. A foot stool is a useful aid. Rest your feet on it when sitting down and place one foot on it while you stand up. Twenty or so repetitions of the angry cat exercise (page 73) each day will help relieve lower backache. If the backache is persistent, a hot water bottle applied to the lower back area can help, as can gentle but firm massage.

You can teach your partner to massage your back during your pregnancy and this will stand you in good stead if you suffer a backache labour. Lie down on your side with your upper leg resting on a cushion or pillow and your back straight. Put some cushions under your head and make yourself comfortable. Ask your partner to place the wide part of his palm between your buttocks and press down hard on the coccyx bone at the base of the spine. Rotate the flesh over this bone, firmly but gently. You may find it helpful to rock your pelvis simultaneously.

For upper back pain and the relief of tension between the shoulder blades, sit on a chair backwards with your arms resting on the back of the chair. Lean forward onto a pillow or cushion. You will probably find this position quite comfortable as it takes the weight of the uterus and baby off the lower back. Ask your partner to massage your shoulders, kneading gently with his thumbs and bringing them up to meet the fingers between the shoulder blades.

When your shoulders feel easier, he should lower his hands and place them on either side of your spine at the bottom. Pressing down firmly, he can then move them right up the spine, one on either side, towards the shoulders in a continuous flowing movement. This upward stroking is tremendously relaxing.

Self-massage

Even if you don't feel tense and have no aches and pains it is still relaxing and soothing to massage your own body. It also helps you to get to know it better and to understand what is happening to you in this final month. Always make sure that you are warm and comfortable before you start. Arrange some cushions on a towel or mat and keep a blanket handy in case you get cold.

Massage is always most effective on bare skin so that the muscles can react. You may find it helpful to sprinkle on some talcum powder first to make the skin more silky; or to use some fragrant oil to enable your hands to move more easily across the skin. You will end up smelling wonderful, too.

Don't hurry the process – put aside plenty of time so that you can really unwind and ease out any tension. If you feel nervous, worried or tense, then practise your conscious relaxation exercises first. You could try closing your eyes while you massage yourself and just concentrating hard on what you are doing and blocking out all other thoughts. You will then be more aware of the sensation of touch and what is happening to your body.

1 Start off with your face and scalp: close your eyes and, with your fingertips only, gently smooth out the skin working outwards from your nose and sweeping up the sides of your face and under your eyes to your hairline. Finish the movement by pressing down into the hollows on either side of your forehead. Repeat several times, starting off from lower down your face – the bottom of your nose, mouth, jaw and chin.

2 Now massage your body: it's best to do this after a bath or shower while your skin is warm and receptive. Make gentle circular movements on either side of your abdomen – don't press too hard. Now when you have established a steady rhythm, start running your hands gently but firmly up over your 'bump' finishing in the centre at the top under your breasts and then stroking back down the sides and underneath. Now just *brush* your fingers backwards and forwards across the skin underneath the 'bump' as though you were stroking the baby inside.

As you get further into your pregnancy you will find yourself tiring more quickly. Take time to relax in a comfortable chair and use these opportunities to catch up on reading, letter writing or having friends to visit. Gentle hobbies such as painting, drawing, sewing and knitting, can be practical and useful, help prevent you from becoming bored and will keep you relaxed and calm.

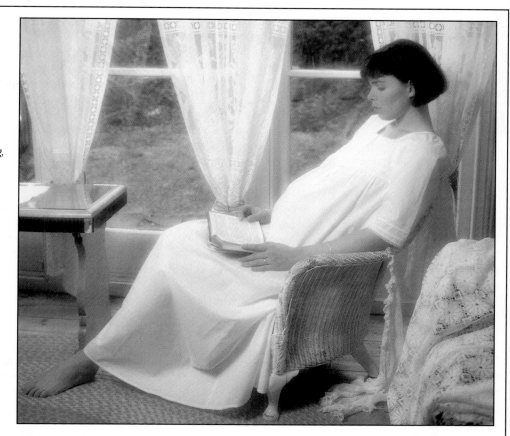

3 Next your neck and shoulders: gently massage the back of your neck and the area between the shoulder blades. Then turn your head to the right and place your left hand on the right side of your neck. Pull it round your neck in one deft movement, gently but firmly, to the front. Repeat on the left side. Massage your right shoulder with your left hand and vice versa to ease out any tension and pain.

Beauty aids for labour

Even when you're in labour, it helps to have some basic beauty aids to keep you feeling cool and refreshed, to relieve backache, to aid massage and generally make the whole experience more comfortable. Many of these items you would probably not think to take into hospital with you but they will be useful when the long awaited day arrives. Don't leave it to the last minute to buy them – you never know when labour may start so keep them ready for a speedy departure.

1 A mineral water facial spray in an aerosol can is refreshing and cleansing during labour when you are feeling hot and uncomfortable. These are available at most drugstores. Alternatively, some 'wet wipes' or soothing eau-de-cologne pads are very cooling and help make you feel less sticky. Just wipe them across your forehead and face, your hands and wrists.

2 A make-up sponge in a vacuum flask of iced water can be squeezed out to cool you down and even used to suck on when your mouth gets dry – you might not be allowed to drink a lot of fluid.

3 Some lip salve in a handy swivel case, or petroleum jelly, will help keep lips moist and prevent any dryness.

4 Soothing, moisturizing body lotion, baby oil or even some fragrant talcum powder are useful massage aids if you experience backache.

5 Some refreshing toner dabbed onto the face with cotton wool pads will make you feel fresher in the early stages of labour.

Of course, it's not a good thing to wear make-up when you're in labour and you certainly won't feel like checking in the mirror on whether your mascara is still intact! However, don't forget to take your cleanser, moisturizer and cosmetics with you. When you're recovered and are ready to receive some visitors, you may feel fresher and better if you just tidy up and quickly repair your face. Even though you will have become a mum, you can still look glamorous!

Nutritious short-cuts to easy meals

During the last month of your pregnancy you probably will not feel like spending a great deal of time in the kitchen cooking, especially if your back and legs are aching. However, it is still very important to eat a high-quality diet and to ensure that your baby gets plenty of nutrients for her growth and development.

Another reason why you should eat well is to build up your strength for imminent labour. In a long labour you will need stamina and endurance and you must prepare for this in the same way as an athlete does for a big race. So don't skimp on your food now or try to start regaining your figure by embarking on a last-minute crash diet. Continue eating a really healthy, nutritious diet but take short-cuts in the preparation and cooking of meals.

For example, you can buy some really healthy convenience foods and ready-cooked meals that only require heating. Many lines and brands contain no additives and are very pure – just look at the labels to be on the safe side. Some supermarket chains make interesting fresh salads in a wide range of dressings, as do many specialist delicatessens.

In supermarkets and health food stores you will see a wide range of convenience and canned foods which, with a little doctoring, can make delicious healthy meals. For instance, you can mix chopped gammon or ham, canned tomatoes and molasses with a humble tin of baked beans and serve with a pre-cooked vegetable dish such as cauliflower cheese, broccoli mornay or a vegetable bake. Most stores sell a varied range of fresh and frozen prepared pasta dishes. Accompany them with a fresh salad.

Of course, there are also takeaway options if you enjoy Chinese food, pizza, curries, hamburgers or fish and chips. Some city-based companies will even deliver the meal to your home – all you need do is pick up the phone and order.

If you have to cook for yourself and your family, then choose simple dishes rather than elaborate gourmet meals. Grilled and stir-fried food is ideal – both quick and easy to prepare and cook so that you spend less time in the kitchen. Make use of any

kitchen aids and gadgets to reduce your labour – use the food processor to chop, slice, grate, mix, or purée. If you have a dishwasher, don't wash up by hand but gradually fill up the machine throughout the day and turn it on while you relax and put your feet up after the evening meal.

You need spend only a short time in the kitchen to make these simple but appetizing dishes.

Moroccan kefta

300g/10oz minced lean lamb or beef
½ small onion, grated
45ml/3 tablespoons chopped parsley
salt and pepper
2.5ml/½ teaspoon each cumin and paprika
1 clove of garlic, crushed
juice of 1 small lemon
Hot sauce:
30ml/2 tablespoons tomato ketchup
15ml/1 tablespoon hoisin sauce
few drops chilli sauce
good dash of Worcestershire sauce

Blend all the ingredients for the kefta together and, with wet hands, mould the mixture around long skewers to about 2.5cm/1in thickness and 7.5cm/3in long. Grill until well browned, turning occasionally. Meanwhile, make the hot sauce (optional) by blending all the ingredients. Serve with brown rice and a salad. Makes 2 servings.

Pasta Napoli

1 onion, chopped
30ml/2 tablespoons oil
2 courgettes, sliced
100g/4oz button mushrooms, sliced
450g/1lb canned tomatoes
15ml/1 tablespoon tomato paste
pinch sugar
5ml/1 teaspoon dried oregano or basil
225g/8oz wholewheat pasta shapes or macaroni
50g/2oz grated Cheddar cheese

Sauté the onion in the oil until soft. Add the courgette and mushroom and fry gently for 2-3 minutes. Add the tomatoes, seasoning, tomato paste, sugar and herbs and bring to the boil. Simmer gently for about 10 minutes until thickened and reduced. Meanwhile cook the pasta in boiling salted water until tender. Drain and serve topped with the Napoli sauce and grated cheese. Makes 2 servings.

Spaghetti alla carbonara

225g/8oz wholewheat spaghetti
100g/4oz diced ham
30ml/2 tablespoons oil
2 eggs, beaten
45ml/3 tablespoons grated Parmesan
45ml/3 tablespoons soured cream or yoghurt
30ml/2 tablespoons chopped parsley

Cook the spaghetti in boiling salted water until tender. Drain and keep warm. Sauté the ham in the oil until golden. Add the spaghetti and stir in the beaten egg. Stir in half the Parmesan and the cream. Season and sprinkle with the parsley and remaining cheese. Serve with a green salad.

Stir-fried chicken and peppers

2 large chicken breasts, skinned and boned
30ml/2 tablespoons sunflower oil
1 onion, roughly chopped
1 large green pepper, seeded
100g/4oz button mushrooms, whole or sliced
150ml/¼ pint chicken stock
15ml/1 tablespoon cornflour
15ml/1 tablespoon soy sauce
15ml/1 tablespoon grated root ginger
2 spring onions, chopped

Cut the chicken breasts into chunks and stir-fry quickly in the oil with the onion until tender. Cut the pepper into chunks and add to the wok or pan with the mushrooms. Stir-fry quickly. Blend a little chicken stock with the cornflour to a smooth paste and gradually add the remaining stock, stirring to eliminate lumps. Pour into the wok with the soy sauce and ginger. Stir until the sauce starts to thicken. Season to taste and garnish with chopped spring onion. Serve with boiled noodles. Makes 2 servings.

Beef Pizzaiola

4 thin slices rump or sirloin steak
30ml/2 tablespoons olive oil

1 small onion, thinly sliced
1 clove garlic, crushed
30ml/2 tablespoons chopped parsley
400g/14oz canned tomatoes, chopped
pinch of sugar

Sauté the steak in the oil with the onion and garlic. Add the herbs and tomatoes, bring to the boil and then cook over medium heat until the sauce is thick and reduced. Season to taste and add a pinch of sugar. Serve with buttered noodles and green salad. Makes 2 servings.

Grilled fish with bananas

2 whole soles, plaice, mullet or bass
salt and pepper
30ml/2 tablespoons olive oil
2 bananas
25g/1oz/2 tablespoons butter
30ml/2 tablespoons mango chutney

Ask your fishmonger to trim the flatfish and remove the heads, or to gut and scale the round fish and cut off the heads. Dust with salt and pepper, brush with olive oil and cook under a hot grill until the skin browns and the flesh turns opaque. Turn and grill the other side. Peel and cut each banana in half lengthways. Sauté in the butter until golden-brown. Heat the chutney. Serve the fish with the sliced banana and chutney. Makes 2 servings.

Tandoori chicken kebabs

juice of ½ lemon
1 small onion, chopped
1 clove garlic, crushed
150ml/¼ pint natural yoghurt
good pinch each coriander and cumin
2.5ml/½ teaspoon curry powder (optional)
salt and pepper
450g/1lb chicken breasts, skinned and boned

Blend the lemon juice, onion and garlic to a smooth paste in a liquidizer or mortar. Mix in the yoghurt, spices and seasoning. Cut the chicken into large chunks and marinate in this mixture for 2-3 hours in the refrigerator. Thread onto skewers and grill until cooked through, turning occasionally. Serve with rice and salad. Makes 2 servings.

Nutritious short-cuts to easy meals

Kebabs

350g/12oz pork or lamb fillet, cubed
juice of 1 lemon
50ml/2floz sunflower oil
2 cloves garlic, crushed
salt and pepper
30ml/2 tablespoons dried oregano
1 small red pepper, seeded
1 small green pepper, seeded
4 rashers streaky bacon
8 large presoaked prunes
1 onion, cut in chunks

Marinate the meat in the lemon juice, oil, garlic, seasoning and herbs for at least one hour. Cut the red and green peppers into large chunks. Remove the rind from the bacon and cut each rasher in half and wrap around a prune. Thread the meat, peppers, prunes and onions alternately onto 4 long kebab skewers. Pour any remaining marinade over the top and grill until cooked, turning occasionally to ensure even cooking. Serve with brown rice and salad or carrot purée. Makes 2-3 servings.

Mushroom salad

45ml/3 tablespoons vegetable oil
450g/1lb button or oyster mushrooms, thinly sliced
1 medium-sized onion, finely chopped
15ml/1 tablespoon freshly chopped parsley
1 cucumber, finely diced
3-4 tomatoes, peeled, seeded and sliced
75ml/5 tablespoon olive oil
15ml/1 tablespoon white wine vinegar
freshly ground black pepper
1 small iceberg lettuce

Liver Veneziana (right) is nutritious and tasty. It makes a filling snack meal and involves very little preparation.

Heat the oil in a large frying pan and gently sauté the mushrooms and onion for 2-3 minutes, or until they are just soft. Allow to cool. When the mushrooms have cooled, stir in the parsley, cucumber and tomatoes. Mix together the oil, vinegar and pepper in a small jug, and pour over the mushroom mixture. Stir gently to coat evenly, and refrigerate for 1-2 hours. Shred the lettuce finely and arrange on a serving plate. Spread the chilled mushrooms evenly over the lettuce.

Liver Veneziana

2 large onions, thinly sliced
45ml/3 tablespoons olive oil
salt and pepper
4 very thin slices calf's liver
few leaves of fresh sage (or chopped parsley)

Cook the onions slowly in the oil until soft, melting and golden. Season to taste. Turn up the heat and add the liver and sage. Fry very quickly – less than one minute each side. Serve immediately with a

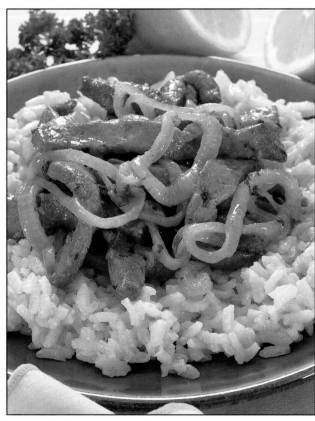

Try some of these healthy convenience meals that are quick and easy to prepare. Mushroom salad tastes as delicious as it looks and Salade Niçoise is a good source of protein and vitamins. Both make wholesome and appetising dishes.

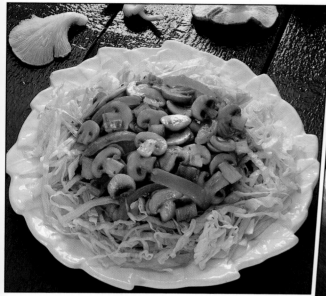

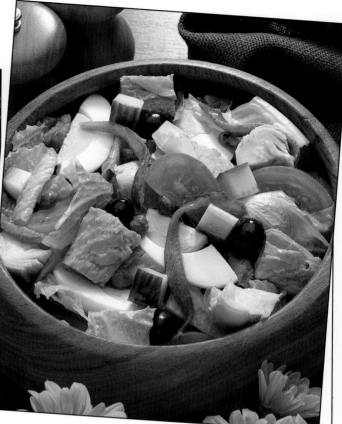

salad of sliced fresh oranges and chopped spring onion, and some brown rice. Makes 2 servings.

Devilled turkey salad

175g/6oz mange-tout
350g/12oz cooked turkey, cut into bite-sized pieces
1 red pepper, seeded and diced
1 yellow pepper, seeded and diced
25g/1oz pine nuts
Dressing:
60ml/4 tablespoons sunflower oil
15ml/1 tablespoon wine vinegar
5ml/1 teaspoon Worcestershire sauce
2.5ml/½ teaspoon paprika
2.5ml/½ teaspoon mustard
pinch of ground cumin
salt and pepper
Garnish:
1 kiwi fruit, peeled and sliced

Cut the mange-tout in half and place in a bowl. Pour over boiling water and leave to stand for 2 minutes, then rinse under cold water and drain. Place in a salad bowl with the other ingredients. Make up the dressing and pour over the salad and toss together. Divide between 4 dishes and garnish with the slices of kiwi fruit. Makes 4 servings.

Salade Niçoise

1 head cos lettuce
2 hard-boiled eggs, quartered
2 large tomatoes, quartered
6 anchovy fillets
10 pitted black olives
15ml/1 tablespoon capers
¼ cucumber, diced but not peeled
1 can tuna fish, drained
4 large artichoke hearts, quartered
Dressing:
90ml/6 tablespoons olive oil
30ml/2 tablespoons white wine vinegar
½ clove garlic, crushed
5ml/1 teaspoon mustard
salt, pepper and lemon juice

Wash the lettuce well, pat dry and break into bite-size pieces. Prepare the remaining ingredients and toss with the lettuce in a large bowl, taking care not to break up the eggs. Mix the dressing ingredients together and whisk until well emulsified. Pour the dressing over the salad just before serving. Serves 4.

Rehearse your positions for labour and birth

It will be helpful during labour if you practise the various positions first so that you can find out which is most comfortable and relaxing. During the first stage of labour, mobility is important and you will probably find it easier to walk about and carry on with things as normal for as long as possible. When you feel a contraction coming on, you can stop and lean against a table or chair or crouch down on all-fours. Some of the positions you can adopt are shown here.

Some hospitals may encourage women to lie down and go to bed throughout the whole of the labour, but it makes sense to stay upright as long as possible so that gravity works with you – not against you – and subsequently your baby's head can press down, the cervix dilates faster and your labour should be shorter. While you are moving around, you boost your circulation in the lower half of your body, too.

Even if you cannot walk around you can kneel or sit propped up so that gravity is continuing to work for you and help your uterus to contract. Trying to function as usual for as long as possible will help dull any pain. You can help yourself by putting off going to the hospital until you feel that it is absolutely necessary. While the contractions are mild and infrequent and until they really get established into a pattern, you can continue with your everyday routine.

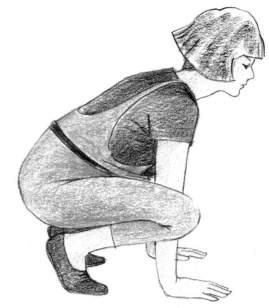

1 Squatting down on your toes and leaning forwards onto your hands for support, can help take the weight off your back. Also it enables you to work with gravity, rather than against it, thus helping your uterus to contract and your cervix to dilate faster. However, this position needs practise as it can be tiring if you are unaccustomed to it, so decide before your labour whether you find it comfortable.

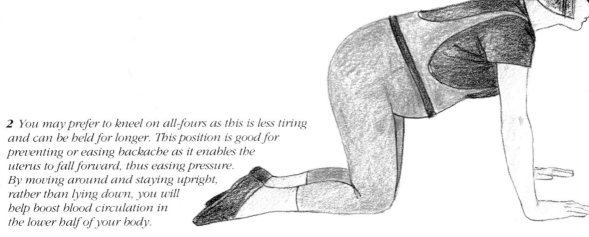

2 You may prefer to kneel on all-fours as this is less tiring and can be held for longer. This position is good for preventing or easing backache as it enables the uterus to fall forward, thus easing pressure. By moving around and staying upright, rather than lying down, you will help boost blood circulation in the lower half of your body.

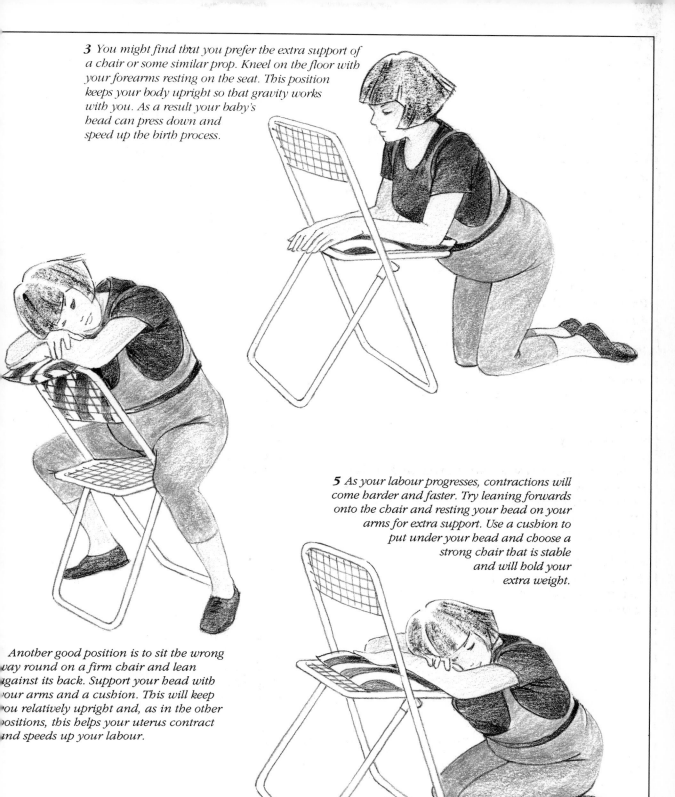

3 You might find that you prefer the extra support of a chair or some similar prop. Kneel on the floor with your forearms resting on the seat. This position keeps your body upright so that gravity works with you. As a result your baby's head can press down and speed up the birth process.

5 As your labour progresses, contractions will come harder and faster. Try leaning forwards onto the chair and resting your head on your arms for extra support. Use a cushion to put under your head and choose a strong chair that is stable and will hold your extra weight.

Another good position is to sit the wrong way round on a firm chair and lean against its back. Support your head with your arms and a cushion. This will keep you relatively upright and, as in the other positions, this helps your uterus contract and speeds up your labour.

Settle into a routine with your new baby

Coming home from hospital with a new baby can be a traumatic experience for many women as they try to establish a new routine, get to know the child and find time for some rest. Unless this is your second child, you are probably unprepared for the time that you will have to spend in looking after the baby – feeding and changing her, bathing and cuddling her, soothing and playing with her. For the first few weeks until she settles down into a routine, it is a full-time job and it is no wonder that many mothers get weary, irritable and even depressed – the so-called post-baby blues.

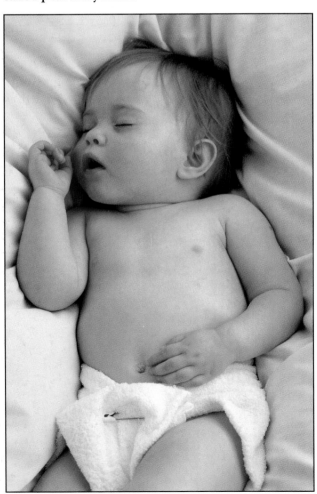

While you are being stretched in every conceivable direction with babycare, possibly looking after other young children, running a home and seeing relatives, friends and neighbours who all want to visit the new baby, you may not have much time left for yourself. But it is very important that you get adequate rest to enable your body to recover from the ordeal of childbirth. You also need to make time for a daily exercise regime to get back into shape (see page 164) and to lavish some beautycare on yourself. After all, you deserve it.

If you had to have stitches, you may feel fragile and rather sore. A warm salt bath twice a day will speed up healing and is a great soother. You will feel refreshed and wonderfully clean afterwards. It may not be possible to have one first thing in the morning and last thing at night – you will have to adapt to your baby's needs and fit bathing and exercising in around feeds. Whenever she falls asleep make sure that you put aside a little of this time for resting and relaxation.

Here is a very brief guide to some of the problems you may encounter with hints on how to deal with them. For more detailed information, refer to one of the excellent books on babycare in your local library or bookshop. However, what follows might point you in the right direction or provide a useful tip for organising yourself better or dealing with a seemingly difficult baby. Let me hasten to add that often the so-called 'difficult' babies who are restless, sleep infrequently and generally make your life awkward turn into the most rewarding children – bright, interesting, active and full of character – so all is not lost and do not despair!

Feeding problems
It is relatively rare for a baby to feed regularly and properly as the textbooks say she should, and most mothers experience some problems to a greater or lesser degree, especially if they are breastfeeding their babies.

Sore breasts can be overcome by applying a specially formulated moisturizing cream available from the doctor or chemist. Most minor sores, inflammations and infections are associated with blocked milk ducts and if you feed the baby gently and often, the duct will soon clear of its own accord.

It will take time for your baby to establish her own sleeping routine. You must be patient and be prepared for some late feeds and broken nights. Also a large part of your time will be spent changing her, bathing her and soothing her.

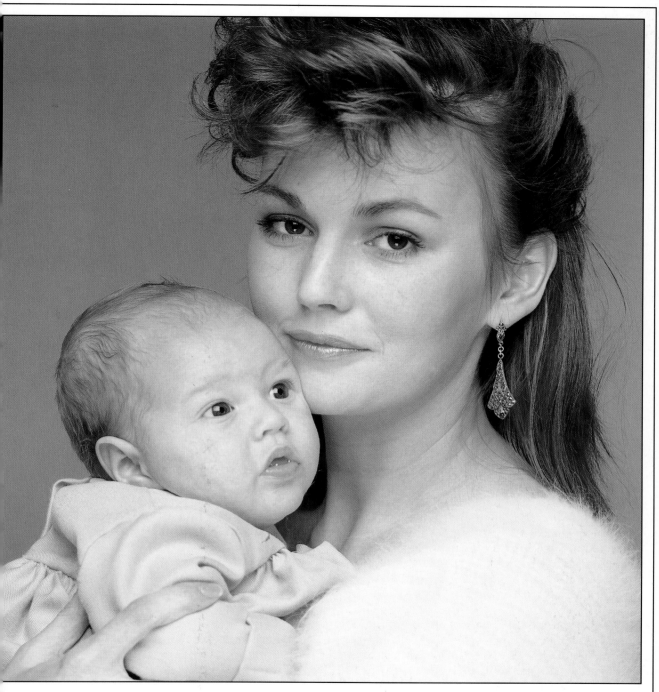

A good varied, healthy diet will help prevent infections and encourage nursing success.

Insufficient milk is another surmountable problem. The baby's sucking action stimulates supply and the more often you feed your baby, the more milk you should produce. Again, if you eat enough high-nutrient foods you should make

When you bring your baby home from hospital, you may initially feel nervous while you learn how to respond to her cries and to look after her. Don't worry as these feelings will soon go as you grow accustomed to your baby's needs.

sufficient milk to satisfy your child. Many women do not persevere at nursing, fearing that their babies are not getting enough milk and that they themselves

Settle into a routine with your new baby

are inadequate in some way for failing to produce it. However, you must bear in mind that breastfeeding may take weeks rather than days to get really established and it is worth persevering for the advantages it brings to you and your baby – more nutritious, anti-infective and non-allergenic milk on tap whenever your baby is hungry. There are *no* bottles to prepare, heat and sterilize.

Your baby is the best judge of whether she has had enough feed. There is no need to limit her to 10 minutes on each breast if she enjoys sucking for longer and finds it comforting, but neither should you sit uncomfortably for hours at a stretch just because your baby likes sucking so much! If the baby looks healthy and content and is gaining weight, then she is probably getting enough milk. However, if her weight does not increase and she cries a lot, you should contact your doctor or clinic immediately and seek expert help. Weighing the baby before and after feeds may be suggested to discover just how much milk she is taking from you. Your local LaLeche League or National Childbirth Trust breastfeeding counsellor will be able to advise you and will be pleased to help. All counsellors are mothers who breastfed their own babies and they will have experienced the problems you are facing. It may be possible to hire a breastpump for expressing additional milk for the baby and to help stimulate the supply if the baby does not like sucking and fails to latch onto the breast properly.

Unco-operative babies are not uncommon and sometimes it takes time to get a baby really hooked on breastfeeding. While some take to it like a duck to water and suck contentedly right from the very beginning, others are less enthusiastic and need coaxing and patience. Give yourself and your baby time to get used to breastfeeding. It is an art *and* a working partnership between the two of you. If, despite perseverance, outside help and advice, your baby still cannot settle down to nursing and it really isn't working, then you will have to introduce the bottle. Do not look on this as being automatically inferior. Neither should you feel guilty about this.

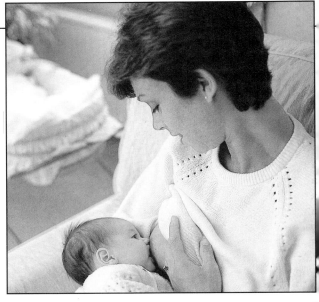

Breastfeeding will give your baby the healthiest, best possible start in life as your milk contains the right balance of nutrients for growth and is anti-infective.

The best way for you and your baby is the one that works and that you both feel happiest about. Your baby will thrive on formula and will feel just as loved, secure and close to you if you hold her tight and cuddle her while you feed her.

Allergies can occur with bottle-fed babies if they are sensitive to formula milk. If your baby is allergic to the standard cow's milk formula, you should substitute a soy-based one instead. Symptoms to watch out for include sneezing, rashes, breathing problems and diarrhoea. Consult your doctor if you suspect that your baby may be allergic.

Coping with a baby
Babies are often incredibly demanding and you will need to work out and establish a system or routine that works for both of you, so that you can enjoy her waking hours, keep her well-fed and clean, and give yourself enough time for rest, household chores, other children, time alone with your partner etc. This is easier said than done and it may be several weeks before you feel really in control of the situation and able to cope with whatever problems arise. Whereas some babies are little angels, sleeping for four or five hours at a stretch and only waking for a feed and changing, others are little devils who rarely sleep and make constant demands on your time.

If you are feeling tired from broken or sleepless nights, a long labour and the unfamiliar stresses of looking after a new baby, it is easy to sink into despondency and feelings of inadequacy. 'I just can't cope' is a common enough cry, especially with first-time mothers who lack the confidence and experience of second- and third-time mums.

If you worked full-time up to the birth of your child and are unused to domesticity and babies, then you may find it doubly hard to adjust to home life and a small baby who is totally dependent on you for all her needs. It can seem very dull indeed just being a mother at home on your own, especially if you had an interesting, creative or stimulating job mixing with many other people every day. A network of supportive family and friends is invaluable at this time, as is an understanding partner. It is also important to be able to escape occasionally for a couple of hours or so and leave the baby with someone you trust.

If you cannot settle down into home routine, you may decide that it is best for both you and the baby if you return to work on a part-time or full-time basis and employ a nanny or a child-minder to look after the baby in your absence. For many career women, this is the perfect solution. They feel happy and fulfilled in their jobs and enjoy their babies even more in the evenings and weekends when they are alone together. In turn the baby may benefit, too, from being stimulated by more than one person, expertly looked after and seeing her mother when she is relaxed and able to enjoy her company and caring for her. A baby may indeed suffer if the mother grows resentful and feels that she has sacrificed herself in some way to stay at home with the child. In my own experience, both my children have been happy with their nannies and have possibly been more independent, resourceful, sociable and less clingy than their peers whose mothers have been full-time house mothers. And you really treasure the time you do spend together.

However, that said, what do you do if your baby falls into one of the following categories?

Sleepless babies may drive you to distraction, especially if they cry a lot. Most babies settle down into a routine within the first month or two, and wide-awake nights soon become a memory. However, there are some babies who do not conform to the hospital routine of four hours' sleep, feeds, change and back to sleep. They seem to thrive on the minimum of sleep and want to play all night, whereas there are others who cry endlessly during the evenings and nights and nothing seems to

comfort them. If your baby falls into this last group, you will probably hear the phrase 'three months colic' mentioned. If your baby seems to be in pain, crying continuously and pulling her knees up into her chest, then she probably has colic.

You can try all the usual remedies – gripe water, winding, cuddling, lullabies, rocking the baby – and yet nothing may have any effect. The important thing is to stay calm and not allow yourself to become irritated, bad-tempered or upset. Comfort your baby – hold her close, cuddle her, feed her and generally just be there to reassure her that you care. You may feel at the end of your tether but remember that she cannot help it (she is not doing it deliberately) and it *will* end. Colic rarely lasts beyond the third month so there is a glimmer of light at the end of the tunnel. Meanwhile, snatch what little sleep you can during the day if necessary.

Reluctant sleepers can be very tired in the evenings but unwilling to go to bed. It is important for both your sakes to try and create a regular sleeping pattern. Put the baby to bed at the same time every night in a warm familiar room. A night light will provide just the right amount of light. A bedtime feed and a lullaby will help the baby to relax into sleep, as can massage. Gently stroke the soles of her feet, her hands, her back and you should feel her relaxing and responding to your touch. Change her nappy last thing just before you put her down. Lay her down on her face or back and tuck her in tightly. Many babies like to be wrapped up and tucked in well and find it comforting – perhaps it reminds them of the womb.

You can have a lullaby music box or even a tape of womb noises to lull your baby into sleep. There are all sorts of gadgets and devices that promise to send babies to sleep. However, there is no magical formula and you must discover yourself what is the best solution for your own child.

If your baby wakes during the night, feed her as quickly and quietly as possible in a dimly lit room. Then, with luck, she will go back to sleep quickly. Unless your baby is upset by a wet or dirty nappy, it is usually best not to change and excite her in the middle of the night but to put her straight back to bed and change her the following morning.

Do not leave the baby to cry for too long before going to her. She will not go back to sleep if she is hungry. Demand feeding is probably the easiest way to cope with these broken nights until the baby establishes her own sleeping routine.

Get back in shape with a work-out

Although you *will* look and feel slimmer, your stomach may be rather flabby and you will have to exercise regularly to tone up the muscles in your abdomen and waist.

Do not be over-eager to get started on your postnatal exercise programme and attempt too much too soon. You cannot launch straight into arduous exercises – they have to be introduced gradually as you get stronger and your body heals. In hospital, you will be shown some exercises to start you off. These will focus on your abdominal, waist and pelvic floor muscles.

Although looking after your baby may not leave you with much spare time for exercise, it is

Getting your figure back

Do not expect your figure to shrink miraculously back to its pre-pregnancy shape immediately after birth. Many women pack a pair of their favourite jeans in a suitcase to wear home from hospital and are horrified when they cannot zip them up.

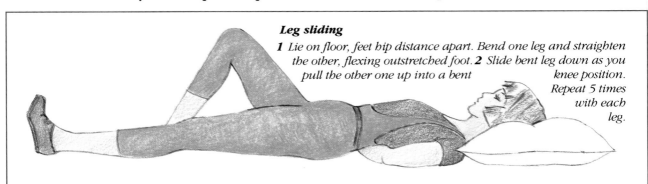

Leg sliding
1 Lie on floor, feet hip distance apart. Bend one leg and straighten the other, flexing outstretched foot. 2 Slide bent leg down as you pull the other one up into a bent knee position. Repeat 5 times with each leg.

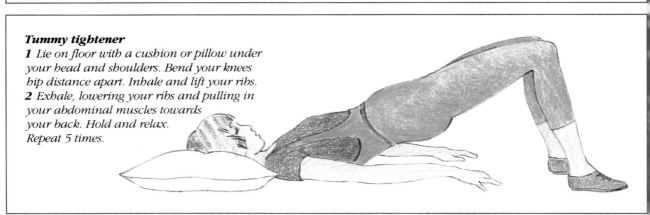

Tummy tightener
1 Lie on floor with a cushion or pillow under your head and shoulders. Bend your knees hip distance apart. Inhale and lift your ribs. 2 Exhale, lowering your ribs and pulling in your abdominal muscles towards your back. Hold and relax. Repeat 5 times.

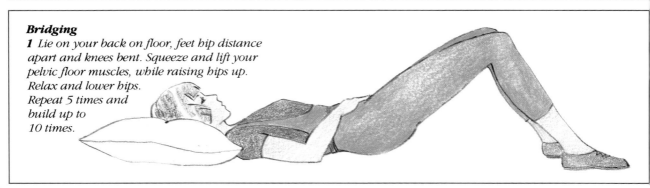

Bridging
1 Lie on your back on floor, feet hip distance apart and knees bent. Squeeze and lift your pelvic floor muscles, while raising hips up. Relax and lower hips. Repeat 5 times and build up to 10 times.

Head lifts

1 Lie on your back, feet hip distance apart and hands clasped behind your head. Bend your knees and keep feet flat on floor. Inhale and raise your head and shoulders off the floor fractionally as you exhale. Only lift yourself as far as feels comfortable. 2 Relax. Slowly build up to 5 repetitions after the second week following your labour.

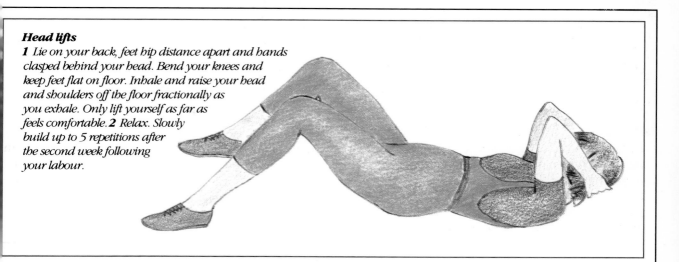

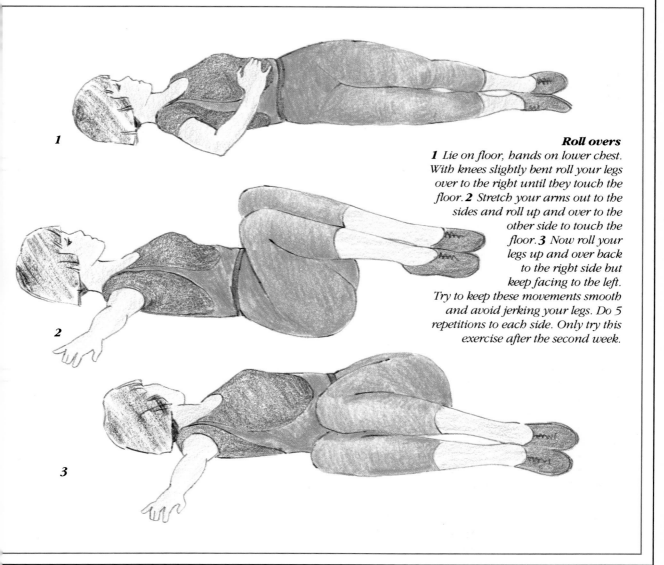

1

2

3

Roll overs

1 Lie on floor, hands on lower chest. With knees slightly bent roll your legs over to the right until they touch the floor. 2 Stretch your arms out to the sides and roll up and over to the other side to touch the floor. 3 Now roll your legs up and over back to the right side but keep facing to the left. Try to keep these movements smooth and avoid jerking your legs. Do 5 repetitions to each side. Only try this exercise after the second week.

Get back in shape with a work-out

important to spend at least 10 minutes a day exercising. Always perform the movements smoothly and slowly without any jerky, awkward movements. Only contract and tighten the muscles for as long as feels comfortable (3-4 seconds is best initially) and then relax. Before exercising, take a few deep breaths and do *only* the recommended exercises.

Remember that your muscles and joints will be weaker than normal for a few weeks after the birth, and you should not attempt any strenuous exercise for at least six weeks. At this stage, you can reintroduce some swimming, cycling or bouts of alternate jogging and walking as well if you wish.

Pelvic floor exercises
It is important to start strengthening your pelvic floor muscles and restore their tone after your baby is born. If you fail to do this, there is always the risk of an inability to hold water or a prolapsed womb in later life. Practise these exercises several times a day, sitting, standing or lying down. Do not worry about your stitches – they won't burst! In fact, exercising the area will increase the blood flow and promote speedier healing. Just squeeze and lift the muscles around the front passage as if you were trying to interrupt a stream of urine. Practise pulling in the muscles around the back passage, too – hold for a count of 3 and then relax. Also practise the pelvic floor exercises that you learnt during pregnancy.

Abdominal exercises
Before you start any abdominal exercises, check for separation of the abdominal muscles. Lie on the floor with your knees bent, feet flat on the ground. Place some cushions under your head and shoulders. Gently press the fingers of your right hand below the navel. You may feel a gap. Inhale and then exhale, lifting your head and shoulders slowly and tucking your chin into your chest. You should feel the muscles on either side of your fingers closing and, hopefully, no more than one finger can remain in the gap. If this is the case, you can start your abdominal exercises as pictured on pages 164-5 and 168-9. A

good exercise to start off with is to lie on your back on the bed. Pull in your abdominal muscles and just lift your head off the pillows. Hold for a count of 3 and then lower your head. Repeat this exercise 5 times.

Back problems after birth
Many women suffer back problems in this postnatal period. Your pregnancy hormones softened and stretched the spinal and pelvic ligaments in preparation for childbirth. It may take five to six months for your back to return to normal and meanwhile you may experience backache where the spine and pelvis join at the sacro-iliac joint. This can be painful, especially when you are sitting in an awkward position for long periods to feed your baby. Finding a comfortable position for breastfeeding can help relieve any backache, as can taking general precautions to avoid pain such as bending your knees when lifting objects, wearing a baby sling that carries your baby centrally and using a pram or buggy with handles at waist level so you need not lean forwards to push it. Never slump in a chair – sit with a supporting cushion in the small of your back and your bottom pressed into the chair-back. The pelvic rocking and angry cat exercises that you learnt during pregnancy may bring some relief.

Postnatal posture
Try to stand and walk tall, tucking in your stomach and buttocks. Posture is as important now as it was during pregnancy. Leaning over to breastfeed your baby and carrying her around can put additional strain on weakened back muscles. If you had a backache labour or an epidural your back may still be sore and painful.

Always make sure that your back is properly supported when sitting down. Put some cushions behind you. Do not stoop or lift heavy objects for the first six weeks after birth. If you must pick something up off the floor or a lower level, bend at the knees keeping your back straight – do *not* lean over. For example, when you lift your baby out of her cot, lower the side and bend your knees to lift her up. Try to change her and bath her at waist level. Put her baby bath or changing mat on a flat surface where you can stand or sit comfortably and avoid unnecessary bending.

Getting enough rest
Put aside some time every day for rest as well as

exercise. The best way to rest in the early weeks is flat on your stomach as this position will help your uterus to return to its pre-pregnancy position. You may feel more comfortable if you support your head and stomach with cushions or pillows. Practise the conscious relaxation techniques as outlined on pages 144-7 so that you are completely rested. Do not feel guilty about putting your feet up like this during the day. Rest will help to make you stronger and enable your body to recover more quickly so that you can resume work or your usual busy routine.

Exercising after a Caesarean birth

Most of the exercises shown are suitable only after a normal vaginal delivery. If you had a Caesarean section, you should ask the hospital physiotherapist which exercises you can do safely. Bear in mind that this is a major operation and it will take time to recover. You will need plenty of rest and relaxation after the birth. You will probably feel really tired and experience some pain. However, you will also want to get to know and look after your new baby and the new relationship between you will compensate for any discomfort you might feel.

If you delivered by epidural rather than by a general anaesthetic, the chances are that you will feel less shocked and nauseous the day after the birth. However, your abdomen *will* feel very sore indeed in the incision area, and you may need painkillers to control the pain and minimize any discomfort.

Breastfeeding may be difficult initially – just getting into a comfortable position in which to feed the baby without causing pain or putting pressure on the incision. Do not be disheartened if everything does not seem perfect straight away. The healing process is going to take time and you must be patient. You must experiment with different ways of lying or sitting to feed your baby. The hospital staff will help and advise you.

The most important exercise you can have after a Caesarean section is to get out of bed and just walk around, however slowly and gingerly. Do this as soon as you can to help avoid any blood clots forming in your legs. Your abdomen will probably feel painful when you walk. Try to brace the area as you move and walk straight and tall – don't stoop. Also try to breathe rhythmically and deeply as you were taught in antenatal classes. Just keep thinking of your wonderful new baby, and the pain can be perceived as worthwhile and a small price to suffer.

It will be several weeks before your wound heals completely and you must not rush into an actively strenuous exercise programme on any account. Exercises have to be introduced gradually as you feel progressively stronger. Holding your abdomen may help you to move more easily and confidently in the early days after the operation.

The first exercises you can practise are the ones for your pelvic floor muscles. Just squeeze the muscles inside you as though you are lifting them. Even though you did not have a vaginal delivery you should practise these exercises every day. After all, these muscles took much of the strain of the baby during pregnancy and they need to be strengthened and put back in their right position.

To speed up healing of the abdominal incision, you should start some gentle exercises within a day or two of the delivery. These will help stimulate blood flow in the area and promote a speedy recovery. You may also suffer from painful and embarrassing gas in the intestines. Walking around the ward and slow deliberate breathing exercises will help alleviate this problem if it occurs.

For a very simple exercise, lie on your back on the bed, knees bent and feet flat on the bed. Inhale slowly and feel your ribs lifting. Now, as you exhale, feel your ribs falling, and tighten your abdominal muscles. Pull them in but only as far as feels comfortable – gently, smoothly and slowly.

You should check with your midwife or physiotherapist which exercises are safe in these early days and how soon you can progress to more strenuous and difficult ones. Do not on any account be tempted to embark on the exercises shown in the colour pictures in this section until you have cleared them with your medical adviser.

Exercising with your baby

Your baby will be quite 'floppy' in the early weeks, and will probably sleep while you exercise. However, by the time she is six weeks old, you can put her in a bouncing cradle and she can watch you exercise. Talk to her while you go through the routine of your postnatal work-out, or play some music. She may wriggle about as though dancing in her cradle. During some exercises, she could be on the floor beside you. She will enjoy watching you and will smile or chuckle while you exercise. As she gets older and develops head, neck and back control, she can even sit on top of you while you practise pelvic lifts and other simple lower body exercises.

Get back in shape with a work-out

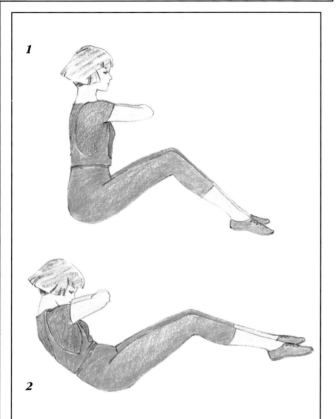

Curl-downs
1 Sit on the floor with your legs stretched out in front of you, knees slightly bent. Cross your arms and hold them away from your chest, lifting your elbows to shoulder level.
2 Inhale deeply then breathe out. As you exhale, lower your chin onto your chest and lean back until you feel your abdominal muscles tighten. Hold this position for a few seconds, breathing normally, then inhale and sit upright. Gradually build up to doing 10 repetitions, taking care not to overstrain. Concentrate on breathing evenly while you are holding this position.

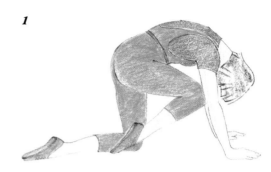

Knee lifts
1 Start on all fours with your knees and hands in line with your hips and shoulders respectively. Inhale. Breathe out and slowly bring your right leg up towards your chest. Try to touch your forehead with your knee.

Curl-ups
1 Lie on your back with your knees slightly bent and your hands resting lightly on your thighs or knees. Inhale. Breathe out and lift your head and shoulders a little way off the ground. Hold for as long as feels comfortable and then gently lower yourself down. Do 10 repetitions. Remember to breathe steadily as you curl up and perform all the movements smoothly and steadily. **2** When this exercise becomes easier, try to progress to clasping your hands behind your head and notice how this increases the stretch in the abdominal region.

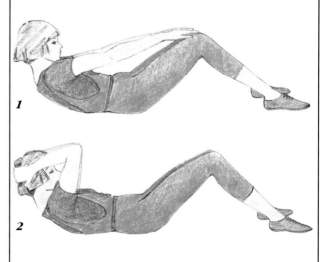

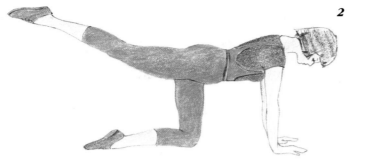

2

2 Inhale again and at the same time lift your right leg up and extend it behind you. Point your toes. Concentrate on keeping your head and spine level, and try not to hollow your back or drop your head down. Do 10 repetitions then repeat the exercise with the left leg keeping all your movements smooth.

Buttock lifts

1 Lie on your back, with your knees bent and your feet flat on the floor. Stretch your arms down by your sides with palms facing downwards. 2 Slowly lift your hips and lower back off the ground until your body is in a straight line from your knees to shoulders. As the hips are raised upwards, try to tighten your buttocks by squeezing together. Hold this position. Relax and repeat 10 times. Try to gradually increase the length of time you hold this lift and feel your buttocks firm up.

1   **2**

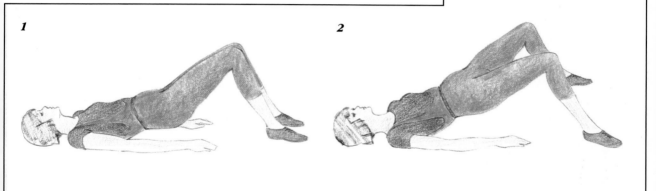

Knee to chest lifts

1 Lie flat on your back with your arms relaxed by your sides. Slowly lift your right leg, bending the knee towards your chest as close as possible. Keep your left leg flat on the floor. 2 Lower the right leg and repeat the exercise with your left leg. Try to keep both feet pointed throughout the exercise and move each leg smoothly and slowly. Do 10 repetitions with each leg and build up to more when you feel ready.

1

2

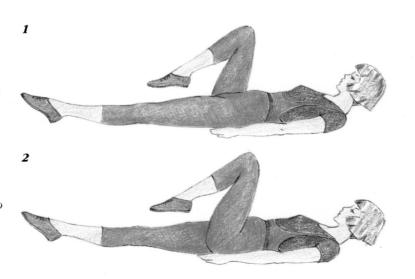

Index

Numerals in *italics* refer to illustrations